Does *My Child* Have a *Speech* Problem?

KATHERINE L. MARTIN

CHICAGO
REVIEW
PRESS

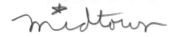

midtour

Library of Congress Cataloging-in-Publication Data

Martin, Katherine L., 1960-
  Does my child have a speech problem? / Katherine L. Martin.
    p.   cm.
  Includes bibliographical references and index.
  ISBN 1-55652-315-7
  1. Language disorders in children—Popular works. 2. Speech
disorders in children—Popular works. I. Title.
RJ496.L35M37   1997
618.92'855—dc20   96-35302
                                                   CIP

Published by Chicago Review Press, Incorporated
814 North Franklin Street
Chicago, Illinois 60610
ISBN 1-55652-315-7
Printed in the United States of America
5 4 3 2 1

5/10/2000 Grad School of Ed & Psych

Does
My Child
Have a
Speech Problem?

Contents

Introduction

As a parent, have you sometimes wondered whether the speech and language development you observe in your child is normal or warrants professional attention?

If certain speech and language behaviors concern you, have you questioned whether your child will grow out of them if you wait long enough or whether there is something you can do to alleviate the difficulties? Or should you be concerned at all? When should you consult a specialist in the area of speech and language, and when should you allow development to take its course?

If you are an educator, what can you do if you observe certain behaviors in the classroom? Has it become tiresome trying to make sense of technical books with no practical approaches?

This book was written in response to the hundreds of parents and educators with whom I had contact as a speech-language pathologist who had similar questions and concerns. I have emphasized the developmental years, which are considered to be the most critical to the successful promotion of speech and language, with practical strategies that can be applied in the classroom as well as at home. This book is not intended to be a panacea for the parent whose child displays severe delays in the areas of speech and language. However, I hope that it will be a resource that both parents and educators can use to make informed decisions that positively enhance a child's development in these areas.

—Katherine L. Martin
Certified Speech-Language Pathologist

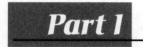

Part 1

Stuttering
and
Fluency Issues

Stuttering defined: A breakdown or disruption in the flow of speech, generally characterized by involuntary or uncontrollable repetitions or prolongations of sounds, syllables, or words.

My child speaks quite well and is very verbal. However, lately I have noticed that he has started to stutter. Should I be concerned?

Many children go through what is called "normal dysfluency," or what some professionals call "developmental stuttering." Fluency refers to how effortlessly a child is able to formulate speech and express himself. Dysfluency refers to a disruption in the flow of speech. When this occurs, speech becomes labored and halting, and the child expends great effort in getting the words out.

Dysfluent periods are typical of children who are experiencing growth in expressive language and speech. As a child's expressive language becomes more complex, sentences become longer, and grammar and vocabulary used are more complicated. As a result, the difficulty in expressing oneself increases. Children are most susceptible to this between the ages of two and six because this is when sentence length and complexity expand rapidly.

Parent Strategy

If a child is going through this period of normal dysfluency, it will generally subside within a reasonable amount of time. There are no hard-and-fast rules, but give your child about six months to work through this stage. However, it would not be unusual if the dysfluency disappeared for a period of time only to recur. If it persists and does not appear to decrease in severity, particularly if the child develops avoidance and fear of speaking situations, you may wish to consult a speech-language pathologist (SLP). And remember, normal dysfluency is not the same as stuttering.

2

How do I know whether my child is a true stutterer versus going through a period of normal dysfluency?

Many factors influence whether a period of normal dysfluency will evolve into true stuttering. Many dysfluent and stuttering behaviors are similar. For example, the child may repeat individual sounds, words, phrases, or sentences in an attempt to speak. Or the child may engage in what are called prolongations: drawn-out pronunciations of words (e.g., "cat" becomes "caaaaaaaaat"). These behaviors are typical of normal dysfluency but can also be the precursors of stuttering.

Evidence of true stuttering occurs under the following conditions:

- Your child does not appear to be outgrowing the problem after at least six months.

- The repetition and prolongation of words become more frequent and intense, with obvious blocks where the child appears to stop in midsentence with facial grimacing in an attempt to push words out.

- The child inserts the "schwa" or weakened vowel into words. For example, a repetition such as "bay, bay, baby" becomes "buh, buh, baby."

- The child experiences an increase in the number of secondary symptoms or behaviors. These might include facial grimacing, loss of eye contact, or excessive tension in the neck and facial area while attempting to speak.

- The child becomes afraid of speaking situations or actually avoids speaking opportunities such as using the telephone, asking for assistance in public places, speaking to authority figures, and so on.

Parent Strategy

Monitor your child for the above behaviors. It is important to remember, however, that all of us at one time or another go through periods of dysfluency depending upon our own level of fatigue, motor coordination, and stress. It is when specific speaking patterns develop and continue, especially if they are extreme, that the parent should be concerned and should consider consulting a speech-language pathologist.

3

If it appears that my child is not going to outgrow a dysfluency or stuttering problem, what can I do?

It would be advisable to seek out the assistance of a speech-language pathologist if the behaviors persist after a reasonable amount of time has elapsed, say six months or so. In particular, this would be recommended if the behaviors are occurring when the child is older (age six and beyond), and if there is a sudden onset. In the meantime, follow the suggestions provided in the Parent Strategy section following, which will aid in reducing the stress for parents both of stutterers and of developmentally dysfluent children.

Parent Strategy

How a parent reacts to the dysfluency or stuttering does make a difference in whether the difficulty improves or worsens. This is not to say that parental reactions create stuttering. However, your reactions to your child's dysfluency or stuttering will influence how your child responds, so it is important to be aware of how you react to the problematic behavior.

Some common parental reactions that should be eliminated immediately include the following (adapted from Zwitman 1978, 29, 30, and 36):

- pained facial expressions
- becoming very still during a stuttering or dysfluent moment
- expressing pity
- expressing guilt over the stuttering
- reinforcing or punishing the stuttering by giving in to requests or withholding rewards, or in some cases spanking the child
- finishing the sentence for your child or filling in with the needed word
- interrupting the child
- asking the child to stop and start over
- telling the child, "think before you speak"
- pretending the dysfluency doesn't exist
- expressing impatience and anger

The following are recommended instead:

1. Listen not so much to the child's speech, but to the content of what he is trying to express. What idea or thought does the child want you to know?

2. Listen calmly and patiently for what your child is trying to say. Resist the urge to jump in and finish sentences and fill in words. Simply say to your child, "I want to hear what you have to say, and we have plenty of time."

3. If your child is in the habit of speaking rapidly, attempt to slow the conversational pace down by waiting before answering. Simply count to three silently before you respond to your child. Don't say to your child, "You're talking too fast." Say instead, "Take your time and go easy. I have time to listen to you." Provide a good role model for your child by monitoring how rapidly you speak.

4. It's one thing to say you have time to hear what your child is saying, but it is quite another to *act* as if you are truly listening. Your child is going to be unlikely to believe you want to listen when you are busy reading a book, watching television, or making dinner. Try to stop what you are doing, get your child's visual attention, and then have the conversation. If it is unrealistic at that moment to drop everything, say to your child, "I really want to hear what you have to say, so let's talk about this in two minutes." Then follow through in two minutes, not ten. Consistency is important.

5. Do not place your child under any unnecessary time pressures to talk. Keep the conversation slow and easy. Many families have a conversational style that conveys a feeling of hurriedness. Try to maintain the three-second rule of waiting three seconds before responding; this will slow the overall pace considerably. Avoid activities that put your child on the spot, such as reciting the alphabet in front of company or having to tell Grandma every detail about what happened in school that day. If the child does not feel like talking, he should not be forced to. Allow him to initiate what he wishes to speak about.

6. Maintain eye contact when your child experiences a dysfluent or stuttering moment. Avoid looking away, looking overly concerned or embarrassed, or acting impatient. Nonverbal communication often speaks more loudly than words. Many parents find it especially difficult to behave the same whether the child is fluent or dysfluent.

7. Be willing to talk to your child about his stuttering or dysfluency concerns when they arise. If the child knows the subject is not taboo, he will likely feel less self-conscious when speaking.

8. Do not interrupt your child. Teach other siblings and family members the rules of turn taking when engaged in a conversation. Neither the dysfluent child nor any other family member should be allowed to interrupt others. Simply state, "Your sister is speaking now, and you may talk without interruption when she is finished."

9. Do not punish your child for stuttering or dysfluent moments. This will only worsen the situation.

4

What role does the environment play in either aiding or hindering the stutterer or dysfluent person?

The environment, both at home and at school, does have an effect on how fluent the child is. The interactions among different members in the family (parents and siblings in particular), the stress level in the home, how family members react to the stuttering behaviors, and overall family conversational styles all influence the child's level of fluency.

Parent Strategy

The speech mechanism is a complex system, and, like most areas of our lives, it is quite susceptible to the effects of our outer conditions. The following recommendations are suggested by Zwitman (1978, 35, 39, 40) to alleviate or reduce negative environmental side effects:

1. Define family rules so that your child knows what is expected of her. Consistency at home is very important:
   - The child should feel that when she begins talking she will not be interrupted, or be allowed to interrupt others who are talking. This applies whether she is dysfluent or fluent.
   - The child should know that when she misbehaves, she will receive a specific punishment that is predictable and noninjurious.
   - The child should know that she will be consistently rewarded for doing her assigned chores.

2. Reinforcement and praise should be used to maintain your child's desirable behaviors and to improve her self-concept and feelings of security.

   - Praise your child for everything she does well.

   - Try to reduce your use of the words "no," "can't," "don't," and "stop it." Instead, make an attempt to tolerate the activity if it is not harmful, or try to redirect the child's interests.

3. Examine your child's schedule. Is there enough free or quiet time?

   - Allow some time every day to spend alone with your child. Fifteen to twenty minutes per day is adequate. During this time, read to your child, take walks, or play. Ask your child *how* her day went versus *what* she did. This enables your child to express feelings more readily.

4. Physical fitness is essential to good speech. Your child must have adequate rest and avoid overfatigue. The more fatigued the child, the more likely dysfluencies will occur.

5. Do not reward the child with sweets. Keep intake of refined sugar to a minimum (e.g., soda, candy, baked goods).

6. Traumatic events such as illnesses, accidents, and emotional conflicts cannot be avoided. Be aware that these events may precede an increase in the frequency of dysfluencies:

   - Accept such dysfluencies as normal given the situation and do not add to your child's stress by reacting to them.

   - Counteract the traumatic event by providing pleasant experiences for your child.

7. Avoid discussing the child's speech in her presence. If your child wishes to discuss it, be empathetic and reassure her that everyone has difficulty speaking at times.

8. Exciting events such as holidays, visits from out-of-town guests, or starting school can result in increased dysfluency in your child's speech. Do what is possible to reduce the intensity of those events.

9. Be alert not only for events but also for people and places that result in increased dysfluency. Change what is possible to enhance fluency.

10. Be aware that your child may become very frustrated if she experiences a great many severe dysfluencies. Provide a way to cope with the frustration, such as:
    - outdoor activity
    - allowing expression of feelings without anyone displaying displeasure or censorship

11. When your child is experiencing a period of increased dysfluency, try to provide successful speaking experiences. Encourage choral speaking (reciting or saying information simultaneously), reciting simple nursery rhymes, singing, and so on.

12. Do not set unrealistic goals for your child. Keep your expectations appropriate for her age level and maturity. Some unrealistic expectations may include:
    - pronouncing words perfectly
    - using an unusually large vocabulary
    - performing difficult motor tasks
    - succeeding in highly advanced academic activities
    - participating in too many activities outside of the home

5

My older child wants to speak for my younger child when he has trouble getting the words out, and teasing is also common. What do you suggest?

It is important to teach siblings as well as other family members that finishing a sentence for the dysfluent child will in no way aid the child. Filling in for the child will only succeed in teaching him that he is incapable of speaking successfully on his own and will undermine the child's self-confidence in speaking. Teasing is not to be tolerated, and parents are encouraged to intervene when this occurs.

Parent Strategy

The following suggestions are recommended by many professionals when a sibling teases the dysfluent child:

1. Take the sibling out of sight and sound of the dysfluent child.

2. Explain patiently and clearly that teasing is impolite and unkind.

3. Discuss the fact that everyone has weaknesses and strengths. Explain that the dysfluent child sometimes makes mistakes when he talks, and that this is no reason to be made fun of.

4. This may need to be repeated several times before the idea gets across. If the teasing still continues, it may be necessary to ask the speech-language pathologist to speak to the siblings.

5. It is likely that, if the child's siblings are noncritical, neighbors, friends, and relatives will treat the child's dysfluencies the same way.

6. The child's teacher may have to handle teasing of the dysfluent child in the same manner if any classmates engage in teasing.

6

If my child is a true stutterer, how will this affect her emotional development and self-concept?

Our own and our children's self-concepts are formulated and affected by those who are closest and most important to us. The expectations, attitudes, and evaluations of those persons will either negatively or positively shape the concept of who we believe ourselves to be.

As stuttering progresses, about the only thing the stutterer can rely on is that the pattern of the stuttering will constantly be in flux. This can create a great deal of stress and anxiety in the child's life. There is an added frustration in that the stutterer does not have total control over when and where an episode of stuttering will occur, whether with a friend or family member, or in a public situation in front of strangers. Unfortunately, many stutterers identify themselves as a stutterer first, and as a friend, sister, or playmate second. Their perceived value of themselves as individuals is often intricately woven into the label of being a stutterer. Much of the research available indicates that stutterers' aspiration levels are lower than those of nonstutterers, not only in speech, but in other areas such as selected vocation, personal goals, and so on (Van Riper 1971, 209).

Parent Strategy

As a parent, it is important to be aware that how you react to your child's stuttering will shape how she feels about herself. You certainly cannot control how society treats the child once she leaves the home environment, but with the assistance of a speech-language pathologist, the child can learn to develop healthy coping patterns when presented with stressful situations. The child must learn that an essential element of healthy coping behaviors is that her own attitude about her stuttering will shape others' attitudes toward her. If the child learns to accept her speaking difficulties with minimal emotional stress, particularly in the form of guilt or shame, it is likely that the listener will be as accepting.

With the assistance of a speech-language pathologist, it is also essential to involve the child's teacher, the family, and significant others in the child's treatment plan. Follow the guidelines mentioned previously, in the answers to questions 1, 2, and 3, when reacting to your child's stuttering. And above all, remember that although you can influence your child's self-concept by how you react to her, do not place the blame on yourself for having caused the child's stuttering. Stuttering is caused by numerous factors that operate together, not a sole etiologic entity. These factors will be discussed shortly.

7

Is there a difference in the occurrence of stuttering in boys versus girls?

Yes. Overall, boys tend to outnumber girls three to one in the general population for a diagnosis of stuttering (Van Riper 1971, 45). There are many theories as to why this is the case.

One theory is based on learning. Most research indicates that girls are more advanced than boys in the early stages of speech and language development. When pressures are placed on both sexes, the likelihood of disruptions in the speech patterns of boys will be greater. It is theorized that boys will be more susceptible to the stress because of their linguistic immaturity. This would also imply that boys may have a less stable neuromuscular control system for speech, at least in the early years.

Parent Strategy

So if your male child starts exhibiting dysfluent patterns, is it automatically assumed that he will develop into a stutterer simply because there is an increased incidence of stuttering in boys? *No.* Boys as well as girls can go through a period of normal dysfluency or developmental stuttering. Follow the guidelines mentioned previously when dealing with the child who is a suspected developmental stutterer, and contact a speech-language pathologist to allay any fears or concerns you may have, particularly if the child does not appear to be overcoming the difficulty.

8

What causes stuttering?

There are many theories as to what causes stuttering, but it would be impractical as well as unrealistic to say that one particular etiology or cause creates the multifaceted nature of stuttering. It is my contention as well as the belief of many professionals in the field that stuttering is a complex conglomerate of internal and external factors and behaviors not easily explained by one simple theory.

Many parents and professionals alike are quite eager to pinpoint any precipitating factors that were present prior to the child engaging in stuttering. Many of the suggested factors have included illness, emotional conflicts, imitating the speech patterns of others, shocking or frightening experiences, or an overwhelming sense of shame or guilt. However, there is much evidence from research that most instances of stuttering began under normal living conditions, with no apparent emotional conflicts present, and under very ordinary circumstances (Van Riper 1971, 87).

Parent Strategy

Take the emphasis away from identifying what caused your child's stuttering, and focus on what you plan to do about it. This will not only help your child, but will also further your understanding of the disorder and how to cope with it. Dwelling on what caused the stuttering is not only wasted energy but is nonproductive. Consult a speech-language pathologist to take the appropriate measures in dealing with the stuttering and your child.

9

Is stuttering genetic?

This is another question that parents often ask. The implication here again is that there must be a deficient gene that is causing the stuttering. It may be safer to say that the research completed thus far indicates a higher incidence of stuttering in families of individuals who stutter than those who do not stutter (Van Riper 1971, 48). However, additional research extending over more than one generation is needed before conclusions can be made as to whether genetic influences are a determining factor.

Parent Strategy

If there is a family history of stuttering, it is again essential that parents do not become overly anxious. A family history of stuttering is no guarantee that the children will be stutterers. Worrying about whether your child will be a stutterer because there is a family history is pointless. If you wish to expend energy productively, inform and educate yourself on what stuttering is. Part VI of this book lists many excellent organizations for anyone interested in learning more about stuttering. Many of our own fears are allayed when we become more educated about what we fear.

10

What can my child's teacher do to assist my child in the classroom, particularly if a diagnosis of stuttering is confirmed?

The teacher's primary task is to alleviate certain situations that can precipitate stuttering. The strategies listed below are strongly recommended for the parent to share with the classroom teacher.

Parent Strategy

Suggestions for alleviating dysfluent speech in the classroom (from an unpublished paper presented by A. Hakanson and J. Wedow entitled "Suggestions for Reducing Dysfluent Behaviors in the Classroom," 1986):

1. Reduce the pressures.
   - Do not place the child under unnecessary time pressures to talk.
   - Do not call on students in alphabetical order so the child will not become nervous as she anticipates her turn.
   - Do not ask the child to recite in class. However, do not single her out as the only one who does not recite.

2. Reduce confusion and indecision.
   - Make instructions clear and repeat them.
   - Minimize speaking in group situations.
   - Set clear guidelines and limitations on assignments.

3. Reduce fear of interruption.
   - Be a quiet, attentive listener, and encourage classmates to be the same.
   - Maintain eye contact when the child is speaking.
   - Do not interrupt or fill in words when the child is stuck on a word.
   - Refrain from detailed questioning.
   - Encourage slow, relaxed talking time for each child where everyone must wait for a child to finish speaking.

4. Limit frustration.
   - Build morale: look for things the child does well, and praise her for them.
   - Create satisfying experiences that bring success to the child.
   - Make the child important and useful in the classroom: give her a job to do that is not intended to be punitive.

5. Reduce insecurity.
   - Be consistent in discipline and praise.
   - Stick to set limitations and rules.
   - Do not draw attention to the dysfluent child by making special allowances for her.

6. Reduce fears of speaking.
   - Encourage participation in minimal speaking situations and show the child that she can get through it. Most children who stutter will avoid speaking situations because they fear they will stutter. Let them know that there will be situations where they will stutter, and that it is OK, and they are still worthy and accepted.
   - Do not tolerate teasing of the stutterer in the classroom or on the playground by classmates. Teach the other children in the classroom tolerance and acceptance of others and what stuttering is: invite the school speech-language pathologist for a class discussion on stuttering.

7. Alleviate maintaining factors in the classroom.
   - Never give the impression that you are anxiously watching the child's speech and are going to change or fix it.
   - Do not show reactions to hesitations or repetitions by the child.
   - Make sure the skills you are teaching are developmentally appropriate.
   - Keep vocabulary usage appropriate, and avoid long and complex sentences.
   - Do not insist on levels of perfection that are beyond the child's capability.
   - Be interested in what each child has to say, and react to what the child says, not how she says it.
   - Do not cut the child off or allow others to do it.
   - Consult with the school speech-language pathologist on a regular basis.

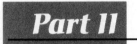

Part II

Articulation Issues

Articulation defined: The ability to speak clearly and intelligibly. Articulation is considered a motor act, meaning that muscle movement is involved. Specifically, articulation involves the actions of the tongue, lips, teeth, and throat to produce the sounds of speech. If a child has difficulty in controlling or coordinating the organs of speech to produce the sounds of her native language, she is said to have an articulation problem or disorder.

11

My child is having difficulty saying certain sounds when he speaks. It is difficult at times to understand what he is attempting to say. What is this?

Your child is experiencing an articulation problem. Articulation involves the integration of several anatomical structures to produce speech, but the primary articulators are the tongue, lips, and teeth. Most articulation problems are due to the inability to place the tongue in the correct position in the mouth or oral cavity. As a result, the speech sounds that are produced are incorrect (see Appendix A).

A common articulation error includes substitution of one sound for another. A child may say "wed" for "red" or "thay" for "say." Another type of error is that of omission. The child may omit a sound when speaking. This can occur in any portion of the word but is most commonly in the final position (e.g., "ba" for "ball"), with less occurrence in the initial position of words (e.g., "all" for "ball"). A third type of error includes that of distortion. The child attempts to make a close approximation of the correct sound but is off target, and the result is indistinguishable to the listener. For example, the child may produce a slushy, unvoiced "l" for "s" in the word "sun." In other words, he substitutes a nonstandard sound for a standard sound.

Parent Strategy

Model correct production of the sound. Do not say "No, that's wrong; say this: _____." Some children need more exposure and ear training than others, and children often need to develop motor coordination of the structures involved in speech production before they become proficient. Simply model the correct production of the mispronounced or misarticulated word, with your face visible to your child.

Create opportunities at story time to select pictures from the book you are reading that contain the sound or sounds that are difficult for your child. Model the correct production of the word, and have your child repeat after you. Do not require perfect production. You simply want to provide exposure to the sound to develop awareness of what he hears and sees when you are producing the sound.

Another awareness activity is to develop a "sound book" for your child. Sort through old magazines and find pictures that contain your child's sound in either the beginning or final position of the word. For example, if your child is having difficulty with the "s" sound, select simple, monosyllabic (one-syllable) words that begin and end in "s," such as "sun" or "bus." Single-syllable words will be much easier for your child than longer, or multisyllabic, words. At first, avoid words that begin with a consonant cluster (such as "stuck," "star," or "smoke"). Also, first develop awareness of words that start with a particular sound, and then proceed to words that end with

that sound. Your child will be more easily able to see you produc
sound if it is in the beginning of the word.

Once you have selected the pictures you want in your sound bo
go through the book and name all the pictures, with your child listening only and watching your face. Randomly point out to your
child where you hear the sound. Using the examples above, you may
say to your child, "Here is a picture of the sun. That word starts with
sssssss" (making a sound like a hiss). Or "This word also has your
sound—busssss." Try to emphasize the target sound. It is also helpful
to make analogies with some children. Say to your child, "This is the
sound a snake makes: ssssssss" or "This is the roar of a lion:
rrrrrrrrrrrr." Always be certain that your face is visible to your child
in any speaking activity.

12

At what age should I expect my child to achieve mastery of most speech sounds? Should I be concerned if she cannot say certain sounds by the time she reaches kindergarten?

Most children master all speech sounds by the age of eight, acquiring
new sounds in a developmental sequence, with the easier sounds
learned before the more difficult ones. The following are average age
estimates of when consonant production occurs (Sander 1972, 62):

"p"	age 1.5 to 3 years	"f"	age 2.5 to 4 years
"m"	age 1.5 to 3 years	"y"	age 2.5 to 4 years
"h"	age 1.5 to 3 years	"r"	age 3.0 to 6 years
"n"	age 1.5 to 3 years	"l"	age 3.0 to 6 years
"w"	age 1.5 to 3 years	"s"	age 3.0 to 8 years
"b"	age 1.5 to 4 years	"ch"	age 3.5 to 7 years
"k"	age 2.0 to 4 years	"sh"	age 3.5 to 7 years
"g"	age 2.0 to 4 years	"z"	age 3.5 to 8 years
"d"	age 2.0 to 4 years	"j"	age 4.0 to 7 years
"t"	age 2.0 to 6 years	"v"	age 4.0 to 8 years
"ng"	age 2.0 to 6 years		

"th"   voiceless, as in the word "<u>th</u>umb" age 4.5 to 7 years

"th"   voiced, as in the word "<u>th</u>at" age 5.0 to 8 years

"zh"   as in the word "mea<u>s</u>ure" age 6.0 to 8.5 years

Thus, the response to this question depends on the age of your child, the sounds that are in error, and whether there are any physical defects present. If, for example, your child is six years old and cannot produce the "s" sound consistently, give her more time to develop this skill before consulting a specialist.

Finally, many parents ask how each sound is produced. The following guide provides a summary of how each sound is created and what articulators or anatomical structures are involved (Newman et al. 1985, 20–24):

Consonant Production and Placement

Stops and Plosives—created from the build-up of pressure and then a rapid release or explosion of air

"p" and "b"
Sound is made by placing the lips together. Air pressure builds behind the lips, followed by a release of pressure and parting of the lips.

"t" and "d"
Tongue tip and blade are in contact with the alveolar ridge behind the upper front teeth, with the sides of the tongue in contact with the upper teeth and gums. An airtight seal is created. Pressure builds within the oral cavity and then is released.

"k" and "g"
The back of the tongue is placed in contact with the velum (back of the palate, or roof of mouth). Pressure builds behind this closure and is released.

Fricatives—created by the flow of air (the breathstream) through a narrow constriction

"f" and "v"
The inner border of the lower lip is raised to the point of contact with the upper front teeth.

"th" (voiced and voiceless, as in "this" and "thin")

The flattened tip of the tongue is placed on or very close to the upper front teeth. Lower teeth are in contact with the undersurface of the tongue.

"s" and "z"

The sides of the tongue are in contact with the teeth and gums. The blade of the tongue is near but not touching the alveolar ridge. A narrow groove is created in the middle of the tongue through which the airstream passes.

"sh" and "zh" as in "measure"

The sides of the tongue are in contact with the upper teeth and gums. The tip and blade of the tongue are raised toward, but do not touch, the alveolar ridge and front part of the palate. There tends to be a protrusion of the lips with these sounds.

"h"

The sound is voiceless and the source of friction with the air flow is at the level of the glottis and vocal cords. Constriction is minimal, however.

Affricates—combine the plosive and fricative characteristics to produce sound

"ch" and "j"

The tongue is placed with the blade and body of the tongue broadly against the hard palate (roof of the mouth), and often including the alveolar ridge. The sides of the tongue are in contact with the upper teeth and gums. The "j" sound is voiced (i.e., the vocal cords vibrate as the sound is produced); the "ch" is voiceless (i.e., the vocal cords do not vibrate).

Nasals—produced by an open nasal cavity during sound production. The nasal cavity is open only when the following sounds are produced: "m," "n," and "ng."

"m"

The lips are closed and the voiced sound travels through the vocal tract and through the nasal cavity. The tongue is generally not involved and assumes the position of the vowel that follows the "m."

"n"

The tip and blade of the tongue are placed on the alveolar ridge with the sides of the tongue in contact with the upper teeth and gums so that air cannot escape through the oral cavity.

"ng"

The body of the tongue is brought into contact with the lowered soft palate (back portion of the roof of the mouth or palate).

Semivowels, Glides, and Liquids—a movement or gliding motion of the articulators involved to produce speech

"y"

The front part of the tongue is raised toward the front part of the hard palate, or roof of the mouth. The glide is made as the tongue moves to the position for the next vowel of the word being spoken.

"w"

The lips are rounded and then move quickly to the subsequent vowel position, creating the glide movement.

"l"

The tip of the tongue is pressed against the alveolar ridge. The tongue is narrowed so that its sides do not touch the teeth toward the rear of the mouth. The "l" is considered to be a liquid.

"r"

The "r" is both a liquid and a glide. Children often have much difficulty producing this sound because of the lack of articulatory points of contact and the involvement of three chamber resonance cavities created when the tongue is in place to correctly produce "r." These vibrating cavities exist in front of the tongue, in back of the tongue, and at the laryngeal pharynx (the back of the oral cavity). In general, a retroflex tongue position is used for "r," meaning that the tongue is bent or curled abruptly backward, with the tongue tip up.

Parent Strategy

Refer to the preceding list if questioning when the development of a specific sound typically occurs. However, I like to advise parents to use caution when using any developmental chart. It is important to understand that these are strictly guides and that all children learn at different rates.

13

When would speech therapy be warranted for articulation problems?

Again, this depends on the age of your child and what sounds are in error. Check the developmental chart in question 12, but also consider these other factors:

- Are there other physical or congenital factors involved? For example, does your child have cerebral palsy, or was he born with a cleft lip or palate? The status of the physical structures involved in articulation (the oral cavity, mouth, lips, tongue, and so on) and the neurological innervation to these structures is essential to development of articulation skills. If your child has a physical, neurological, or other impairment, early intervention is a must.

- How many of your child's speech sounds are in error? The more sounds in error, the greater the likelihood that your child may need remediation. If your child is misarticulating one or two sounds versus five or six, this is a less serious problem.

- How intelligible is your child's speech to either the familiar or unfamiliar listener? If you cannot understand what your child is saying, chances are that others who are unused to his speech will be equally confused. The more unintelligible your child's speech is, the more likely your child will need professional assistance.

Parent Strategy

Consult a speech-language pathologist (SLP) for an articulation screening if any of the factors above are of concern. In the meantime, follow the suggestions given for development of sound awareness in question 12, and encourage your child to speak at a slower rate to aid in intelligibility.

In the event your child starts speech therapy, many parents wonder what to expect and at what level they can become involved. An SLP will initially begin treatment by teaching the child the sound in isolation first. For example, if the sound in error is the "s," the SLP will begin by modeling the sound and instructing the child where to place the tongue during production. In addition, the child may be given several activities to improve visual, tactile (touch), and auditory (listening) feedback to help him produce the sound correctly and to monitor it for himself.

Once a child is able to produce the sound consistently in isolated form, the sound is then paired with a vowel to form a CV (consonant-vowel) combination. So in the above example with "s" as the target sound, the treatment would focus on combinations such as "so," "see," "saw," and so on. VC (vowel-consonant) combinations would be next. Once the child has mastered this level, treatment then proceeds to words that begin and end with consonants. Monosyllabic (single-syllable) words are generally selected because these are the least difficult. Words that begin with the target sound are selected first, such as "sun," "sat," or "sip." Then once the sound is mastered at the beginning of the word, words are selected that have the target sound at the end of the word (such as "bus," "miss," or "pass.")

When the child has mastered the word level, treatment then proceeds to phrases, sentences, and eventually conversation. This method is generally known as the traditional approach to treatment of articulation difficulties, and not all SLPs use this technique. For example, a condition known as developmental apraxia of speech generally manifests itself as a severe articulation disorder and responds more favorably to nontraditional treatments.

At what level can parents become involved in their child's treatment plan? I highly recommend that all parents work with their children in developing general sound awareness (see question 11), sound discrimination (see question 19), and taking advantage of all visual cues (using a mirror while repeating words in the sound book, watching parental facial features while reviewing sounds or words, and so on). If a child is in speech therapy, I generally do not give actual "homework" for the parent and child until the child has mastered the sound production at the isolated and syllable level.

When therapy has progressed to the word level, flash cards can be developed for home use for the parent(s) and child with words containing the target sound in the beginning position first. But until that stage is attained, development of awareness and selective discrimination is essential. As a last caution, do not attempt to be your child's speech therapist. Consult a certified speech-language pathologist who is licensed, has a minimum of a master's degree, and holds the certificate of clinical competence (CCC) from the national organization (ASHA). See the Closing Remarks at the end of Part V for more information about choosing a speech-language pathologist.

14

I have a newborn baby. What sounds will be the easiest for her to develop first?

The sounds that are the most easily acquired are those that are the most visible when spoken. These sounds include the bilabials (sounds produced with the lips) and include "p," "m," "b," and "w." Less visible but produced earlier are the lingua-alveolars (such as "t," "d," and "n") and glottal sounds ("h"). Lingua-alveolar refers to the contact of the tongue against the alveolar ridge (behind the upper teeth), and glottal refers to the actual opening between the vocal cords at the laryngeal level (the glottis).

Parent Strategy

During the first year, children acquire a phonological system that progressively becomes more complex, starting initially from vowel-like sounds to consonant-vowel (CV) or vowel-consonant (VC) combinations. Definable CV or VC combinations (such as "baba" or "dada") usually don't occur until about the age of seven to ten months, with the first real words appearing at approximately ten to fourteen months. It is at this stage, when the first meaningful words are spoken, that the child will start to acquire the sounds of the language.

To stimulate vocal play in infancy, take your infant's lead. By repeating the vocalizations your infant produces, you are encouraging more vocalizations, which is essential not only to phonological development, but also to language development. Encourage vocal play that includes the more visible sounds first, such as "p," "m," "b," and "w." These sounds can also be readily felt. If you place your infant's hand over your mouth while you say the sound, she will get the tactile feedback while receiving the visual and auditory cues for the spoken sound.

What causes articulation problems?

Most articulation problems can be classified as either organic or functional. When a structural deformity or physical problem contributes to the articulation error, the cause of the problem is organic. An example of this would be an unrepaired cleft lip or palate.

When all observable physical structures appear to be intact (such as teeth, lips, palate, and tongue), as well as the neurological innervation to these structures, the articulation problem can be considered functional in nature, and thus attributed to faulty learning of the sound or sounds.

Parent Strategy

All children go through a developmental period of producing incorrect sounds. If your child still makes these incorrect sounds when it is no longer developmentally appropriate, and if the incorrect sounds are made frequently, then professional intervention is warranted. If there is an organic source to your child's articulation problem (i.e., a physical defect), take measures to remediate this as soon as possible, and enlist the assistance of a speech-language pathologist for articulation remediation. If the cause appears to be functional, consultation with a speech-language pathologist is advisable.

Is it normal for my child to confuse sounds that appear similar in tongue placement or that sound alike?

Every child and her articulation patterns differ, but generally children confuse sounds that have the most features in common and thus sound similar. For example, when substitution of one sound for another occurs such as a "t" for a "d" or a "t" for a "k," the following may be happening:

1. The "t" and "d" sounds are both made with the tongue placed forward in the mouth against the alveolar ridge behind the teeth, with a short explosion of air. However, what distinguishes these as different sounds is the voicing. When you say "t," place your hand lightly over your throat. You will not feel any vocal vibration. But when you say "d" with your hand over your throat, you will feel the vocal vibration. This means that the "t" is voiceless and the "d" is voiced. A child making this type of error has the tongue placed in the correct area but doesn't yet have the concept of a voiced or voiceless sound. The same could be said for substitution of a "p" for a "b," "k" for a "g," "f" for a "v," or "s" for a "z."

2. When the "t" is substituted for the "k," the "t" and "k" are both voiceless and are produced with a short explosion of air. However, the tongue is placed forward in the mouth for "t," but farther back for "k." This is what is commonly referred to as a placement error.

Parent Strategy

These are only a few examples of the types of articulation errors seen and the reasons why they occur. It is essential to stress that every child's speech patterns are different, so acquisition of sounds among different children will vary. Children need frequent exposure from adult models in the form of auditory input (listening to sounds and words), visual input (seeing the words or sounds being produced), and tactile input (feeling or touching the mouth or throat area) to develop an efficient articulation system. Do not demand correct production from your child every time she speaks. Simply model the correct production as mentioned previously, and develop sound awareness (see question 11). If your child's problem requires therapy, work closely with your therapist on a home program for parents that is specific to your child.

17

My child had PE (patent eustachian) tubes placed within his ears as an infant because of frequent ear infections. I am concerned about the effects this may have on his ability to develop articulation skills. What is the relationship between articulation development and middle ear infections?

Otitis media, or middle ear infection, can occur at any age, but primarily affects children from infancy up to age six. Either or both ears can be affected. Some children have chronic infections in one ear. Others experience infection in alternate ears, or in both simultaneously. When the middle ears become infected, fluid accumulates and can often cause great pain and pressure. Chronic and recurrent middle ear infections can create a threat of perforation to the tympanic membranes (the eardrums) because of buildup of pressure in the middle ears from fluid accumulation.

The eustachian tubes are air canals that connect the middle ear to the back of the throat or laryngeal area. They are responsible for equalizing the air pressure in the inner ear to match that in the outer ear or external auditory canal every time we yawn, swallow, sneeze, or change altitudes, as when we travel in a plane or drive into the mountains. They also drain any fluids that have accumulated in the middle ear due to a cold or upper respiratory infection, at least in adults. Middle ear infections are common in young children and infants because their eustachian tubes tend to be shorter, wider, and lying in a more horizontal plane than is usual in adults. As the child grows to adulthood, the eustachian tubes elongate and assume a more vertical position, so that drainage in the middle ear becomes easier.

If a child is susceptible to middle ear infections, the physician, generally an otologist (ear specialist) or an ear, nose, and throat specialist (ENT), will perform a myringotomy (an incision in the eardrum) to relieve the pressure and drain the fluid, and then place PE tubes through one or both tympanic membranes. These small plastic tubes will allow for continued drainage of the middle ears and later equalize the air pressure within the middle ears just like the natural eustachian tubes (Martin 1975, 247).

The tubes can remain in place anywhere from several weeks to several months, after which time they will naturally work themselves out of the eardrums into the external ear canals. Antibiotics are also usually prescribed.

Whenever a child's middle ears are full of fluid, the child will experience a conductive hearing loss—a blockage in the transmission of sound waves to the inner ears, so that all noises and speech will sound muffled. (See Appendix B.) As a result, your child may not be hearing much of what is said to him, or the information that does get to the inner ear may be distorted or muffled. When this occurs, the child will model his speech patterns according to what he *thinks* he hears. If you say "sun" and it sounds like "thun" to your child, chances are that he will say "thun."

A conductive hearing loss is generally temporary and alleviated once the fluid is removed. However, if a child learns a habitual pattern of substituting "th" for "s" or any other errors, he will have to relearn these articulation patterns. The errors won't simply disappear when the fluid is removed.

Note that simply because a child suffers from an occasional middle ear infection, this will not mean that he will automatically have poor articulation skills. It is when the ear infections become chronic that concerns about articulation arise. Research completed by Shriberg and Smith (1983, 294) concurs with this theory. The authors speculate that inconsistent auditory input due to fluctuating hearing losses accompanying middle ear involvement may negatively affect the child's ability to establish underlying features for consonant production.

See question 38 for more information about how otitis media can affect other aspects of language development.

Parent Strategy

Consult your pediatrician or an ear, nose, and throat specialist (ENT, or otorhinolaryngologist) if you suspect a middle ear infection. Immediate treatment is essential to prevent possible perforation of the eardrums and subsequent damage to surrounding structures and tissues. If your child has a history of repeated ear infections, it may be advisable to have his hearing screened periodically by an audiologist.

A consultation or screening by a speech-language pathologist may also be necessary.

18

Please explain the relationship between dentition and articulation errors. Can tooth loss have an effect?

Although a loss of dentition (teeth) can affect articulation, malocclusions have a greater effect. Occlusion refers to the relationship between the upper (maxillary) and lower (mandibular) teeth when they contact one another. A malocclusion is an abnormal occlusive pattern, or relationship, between the upper and lower sets of teeth. In a normal occlusion, the upper central incisors (the front teeth that we typically use to bite into something) extend just slightly over the lower central incisors about one-fourth of an inch. However, in reality, normality is measured by the relationship between the upper and lower molars (back teeth).

The malocclusive patterns that create the most problems in articulation are the anterior crossbite (in which the lower teeth are wider or on the outside of the upper teeth when upper and lower teeth are in contact) and an open bite pattern (where there is a gap between the biting surfaces when upper and lower sets of teeth are placed together). Malocclusions typically affect the fricative sounds, particularly the "s" and "z."

Articulation can be temporarily impaired if some teeth are missing, particularly the frontal incisors. The sounds most generally impaired are again the "s" and "z" sounds, as well as the "th" and "sh."

Parent Strategy

If concerns arise in regard to articulation and you suspect that either dentition or a malocclusion is a contributing factor, consult a speech-language pathologist for an articulation screening and oral-peripheral exam. An oral-peripheral exam is a routine check of the oral structures (teeth, occlusive pattern, tongue, and so on).

19

My child is four and attends a day-care center. His primary companion is a child who has difficulty saying certain sounds. I am concerned that my child may start imitating his friend. Will this happen?

Children certainly do learn speech patterns by modeling or imitating other children and adults around them. But it is essential to remember that your child is in more than one environment each day other than day care, and these environments are equally influential. If your child is not displaying articulation problems outside of what is expected for his age level, I would not be concerned.

Parent Strategy

Develop your child's ability to discriminate and detect correct versus incorrect articulations. Play word games in which you randomly select objects or pictures around the house. For example, if you had a cup on the table, you might ask your child, "Listen. I am going to say the name of this. Tell me if I said it right." Then name the cup as a "tup." Have your child tell you a simple "yes" or "no" if the word sounded right. Then proceed around the room randomly choosing different objects, saying their names correctly at times and incorrectly at others. Change only the first letter in the word initially. Thus, if you had the words "red, coffee, pan, thumb," you could change these to "wed, toffee, ban, sum." This activity aids in discriminations of sound and helps children to develop self-correction and self-monitoring skills that are necessary to articulation development. The game is most suitable for ages four through eight, and the idea is to develop discrimination and listening, so do not require your child to repeat correct productions after you.

20

What is the relationship between articulation skills and a sensorineural hearing loss?

When a child has been diagnosed with a sensorineural hearing loss, this implies that there will be a permanent loss of sound sensitivity and hearing acuity. This is generally because of an abnormality in the inner ear or the nerve pathways beyond the inner ear to the brain.

As a result, the information or speech that is sent to the hearing-impaired person will be affected depending on the severity of the loss. In general, the severity of hearing loss is measured by:

- the loudness levels at which the individual can hear information, measured in decibels (dB)

- the frequencies or pitches that can be heard, measured in cycles per second (cps) or hertz (Hz)

For example, when an audiologist tests a child's hearing, the child may be hearing sounds in the lower frequencies but have a hearing loss in the higher frequencies.

So why do decibel and frequency levels matter in articulation development? Primarily because each consonant or sound has its own decibel and frequency level at which it is typically produced. The accompanying diagram is an audiogram—the chart used to depict a person's hearing abilities—with each consonant charted according to the frequency and decibel level at which it is commonly heard.

For example, if a child had a 60 dB sensorineural hearing loss (no sound is detected below 60 dB) between the 2,000 to 6,000 Hz frequency range, she would have difficulty hearing the following sounds: "th," "s," "f," "t," and "k." Because most consonants are produced between 250 to 2,000 Hz and below 50dB, a sensorineural hearing loss within those parameters would be detrimental to speech and articulation development. You can also see now why a conductive hearing loss would affect articulation skills.

Parent Strategy

If you suspect a hearing loss, have an audiologist evaluate your child's hearing as soon as possible. Refer to the materials in Part VI for home language and speech programs. Contact with a speech-language pathologist will also be necessary.

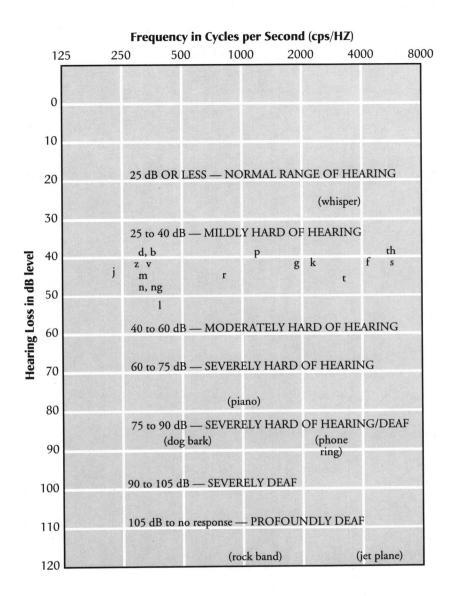

Frequency in Cycles per Second (cps/HZ)

| | 125 | 250 | 500 | 1000 | 2000 | 4000 | 8000 |

Hearing Loss in dB level

0
10
20 — 25 dB OR LESS — NORMAL RANGE OF HEARING
(whisper)
30 — 25 to 40 dB — MILDLY HARD OF HEARING
40 — d, b ... p ... th
z v ... g k ... f s
j ... m ... r ... t
n, ng
50 — l
60 — 40 to 60 dB — MODERATELY HARD OF HEARING
70 — 60 to 75 dB — SEVERELY HARD OF HEARING
(piano)
80 — 75 to 90 dB — SEVERELY HARD OF HEARING/DEAF
(dog bark) ... (phone
90 — ring)
100 — 90 to 105 dB — SEVERELY DEAF
110 — 105 dB to no response — PROFOUNDLY DEAF
(rock band) ... (jet plane)
120

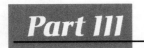

Part III

Listening and Auditory Processing Skills

Auditory processing defined: Auditory processing refers to our ability to listen, accurately comprehend, and respond to information spoken to us, from the initial detection of sound or speech by the external ear to the transmission of that sound via the auditory pathways to the brain.

21

I know my child hears me when I tell him to do something, but it is as if he is not listening. Does he have a hearing loss?

If you suspect that your child is not hearing properly, it is always advisable to have an audiologist test his hearing to rule out any conductive problems (any blockage in the middle or outer ear) or any sensorineural loss (nerve damage); see Appendix B. However, just because a child is not "listening" or following through on instructions does not necessarily mean that the child has a hearing loss.

If the results from a hearing test come back with no indications of any problems with the hearing mechanism (the outer, middle, or inner ear functions), then your child may very well have a central auditory processing deficit. Auditory processing deficits can affect children in the presence or absence of a peripheral hearing loss, and it is important to make the distinction that "hearing" sounds, speech, or noises is different from actually "perceiving" or processing the information heard.

Parent Strategy

If you suspect that your child is having difficulty either hearing or perceiving what is said to him, it is always best to have an audiologist test your child's hearing to rule out a peripheral hearing loss. Then consult a speech-language pathologist (SLP) for an assessment of auditory processing skills. In my experience, auditory processing abilities are one of the most overlooked areas in the field but have the most significant impact on language and academic development in children. Have a proper diagnosis by a speech-language pathologist if you suspect an auditory processing disorder.

22

What is the difference between hearing and auditory processing?

To overgeneralize, when you speak to your child, the information first reaches the outer ear, and the sound is then channeled through to the middle ear (the site of ear infections and fluid accumulation). The information is then transmitted to the inner ear, where the signal is passed to the auditory nerve—the pathway to the brain. Once the signal reaches the brain, the listener then perceives the message or information sent. The "hearing" mechanism primarily refers to the peripheral or outer structures and involves the outer, middle, or inner ear, from which information is then sent via the auditory nerve to the brain.

The processing of auditory information involves the actual perception and attachment of meaning to the signal or sound. When the signal leaves the inner ear and travels up the auditory pathways to the cerebral cortex of the brain, we can then attach meaning to the signal that was heard. Therefore, if there are any problems processing information, they generally occur after the signal has left the inner ear. The breakdown in processing can occur when the signal travels the auditory pathways to the brain, or at the cortical level once the information reaches the brain. As a result, it is quite common to have no hearing loss at the peripheral level (in terms of hearing acuity for different frequencies at varying decibel levels), but difficulty in perceiving or understanding information spoken by others.

Parent Strategy

It is very easy for parents to become quite frustrated when it appears that their child is purposely not listening. However, upon further examination, it may be that the child is listening to the best of her abilities, but the information is getting lost as it travels from the inner ear to the brain. Whether a child has an auditory processing disorder or not (in the absence of a hearing loss), it is essential for parents to modify their behaviors when speaking to such a child. Some of the important considerations include:

1. *Get your child's visual attention first.* Gently touch her arm and say "Look at me. Listen." Then proceed to speak to her.

2. *Minimize the distractions.* Turn down the television, radio, or any noisy appliances before you speak to your child. Background noises will compete with what you are trying to say, and it will be difficult for your child to filter them out.

3. *Stay physically close to your child while speaking.* Don't expect your child to get everything you said the first time if you are in the kitchen washing dishes and she is in the next room watching television, and you tell her to do something and she responds with "What?!"

4. *Monitor the length and complexity of what you say.* A one-part command will be much easier to follow than a three-part instruction. Also, you can ask your child to do something with fewer words and less complexity and accomplish the same end. For example, you could say, "Go upstairs to your room and put all your toys away, all the ones that are all over the floor, and after that wash

your hands carefully in the bathroom, make sure they're good and clean, and then come down and set the table. Dinner's almost ready." However, you could make this same statement but reduce the length and complexity, while retaining the meaning. This is done by selecting the key elements in the message. Thus, the same instruction could be said this way: "Listen carefully. Put your toys away, wash your hands, and set the table." If your child fails to follow a three-part instruction, drop the commands to two parts. If two-part commands are difficult, reduce the command to one part. It is important at all times to be in tune with your child's processing level, and follow her lead.

5. *Increase comprehension through nonauditory communication.* If your child has difficulty processing information in the auditory mode, any means to a different channel will be helpful. As you are telling your child what to do, try augmenting your statements visually. For example, a parent may have difficulty getting a child to follow through on routine chores around the home without having to repeat daily what is expected. In this instance, a chart could be made up with pictures of key items to be processed. Thus, if it is necessary for the child to make her bed, brush her teeth, and feed the dog each morning, the parent could make up one column with a picture of the sun, and in this column place pictures of a bed, a toothbrush, and a dog. For evening chores, make another column with the moon or stars, and put appropriate pictures of the expected activities here. Then as you tell your child what is expected, have the chart in front of her as a visual reminder.

Finally, if you can visually demonstrate activities after telling your child what to do, this can also be helpful, particularly when there is a new task with multiple steps being learned. For older children, it is helpful to write information down in smaller steps, especially if you are attempting to explain a more involved and detailed concept. A tape recorder in the classroom is helpful for middle and high school students, particularly if the material being presented is primarily lecture with few or no visual diagrams.

23

What types of behavior are typical of children who have auditory processing deficits?

One of the most commonly expressed frustrations of parents is that their child "just doesn't listen." Parents often report that they have to repeat information over and over for their child to understand what is spoken, or that they have to oversimplify what is said. Another common complaint is that the child lacks concentration and attention to tasks, particularly in the presence of background noise. Finally, a parent may observe that the child processes all the different parts of the message but gets the information confused and out of sequence.

Although much of the literature has focused on processing patterns in adult aphasics (that is, adults who have lost language ability due to brain injury), I have found that Brookshire's research is quite applicable to the younger population. Children's auditory processing patterns can take various forms, but in general a child may exhibit any of the following patterns (Brookshire 1974, 3–16):

Retention deficit: The child's processing of information decreases as the length of the stimulus increases. For example, it would be more difficult for the child to follow through on a two-part command containing ten words than a two-part command containing six words. Length is the critical issue rather than complexity of command.

Information capacity deficit: The child has difficulty receiving and processing the incoming message simultaneously. For example, when told something, most of us are thinking and formulating ideas about what the speaker is saying as we engage in conversation. Children with this type of deficit often need a time lag between when they receive the information and when it is processed, allowing them to draw their own meanings and conclusions.

Noise build-up: The child's performance worsens as more information is given. Children with this type of difficulty often process information given to them in the initial stages, but as the conversation ensues and complexity builds, it is as if the child's processing system goes into overload and shuts down.

Slow rise time: The child receives the last part of the message but loses the first part. In this instance, it is as if the processing system needs time to warm up before it is ready to receive information.

Intermittent auditory perception: The child's processing system fades in and out. As a result, the child receives bits and pieces of information, and thus any incoming information does not make sense to him. The child responds with either no response, a bizarre response, or a partial response.

Parent Strategy

The parent can respond to the situation on the basis of the predominant pattern exhibited. Here are some suggestions:

Retention deficit: Since length is the critical element here, simply shorten the length of the sentence or instruction given. However, also monitor the complexity.

Information capacity deficit: Allow the child enough pause time to receive the information and then process it. Many children are quite competent if given the time and opportunity to process and formulate their response. It is a good rule of thumb to allow at least eight to ten seconds to pass before repeating the information. This may seem like an interminable amount of time to adults, but to the child who requires the additional processing time, it can mean the difference between success and failure.

Noise build-up: Often the rate of the noise build-up is related to the complexity of the language used. When speaking to your child, monitor the complexity used (such as multiple-level commands, complex details and concepts) but teach your child to stop the speaker when he senses that he is losing what the speaker is saying. In this way, the child is in control of the situation and will feel ready to continue when his system is no longer in overload.

Slow rise time: Children with this type of difficulty need to be readied before they are prepared to receive information. Cues are essential in these situations. For example, physically touch your child's hand or arm, get his visual attention on your face, and say, "Look here. Listen. Get ready. Watch what I say." Then say the message. In this way, if the child misses the first part, he will likely miss the readying cues rather than the content of the spoken message.

Intermittent auditory perception: Children with this type of difficulty may appear to be "spacing out" periodically. When this occurs, get the child back to the present by stirring him into action physically. Have him change his body position, move into a different chair, stand up, and so on. This will aid him in breaking out of the trancelike pattern and getting back on track. However, this type of behavior can sometimes signal a more serious medical condition, such as epilepsy or seizures. Consult a neurologist or your pediatrician immediately.

24

If my child has an auditory processing difficulty, does this mean that she has attention deficit disorder?

Attention deficit disorder (ADD) is a diagnosis that can be made only by a team of qualified professionals including but not limited to a physician, an educational diagnostician or psychologist, and a speech-language pathologist. If a child has been diagnosed with ADD, the condition can often be improved with medication.

ADD is not synonymous with auditory processing disorders. A child who has been diagnosed with ADD generally has auditory processing deficits as one of the many symptoms of this disorder. But if your child has been diagnosed with an auditory processing disorder, this does not mean that she has ADD. Many children and adults have auditory processing deficits without having ADD.

Parent Strategy

If you observe a severe auditory processing deficit in your child, this may signal a more serious problem that can be a possible indicator of ADD. Some behaviors include:

■ difficulty keeping full attention on a task

- difficulty keeping still long enough to process any information or instructions
- difficulty understanding lengthy or complex information
- easily distracted by background noise, outside noises, or movements
- high activity level

If you suspect ADD, a proper diagnosis must be made by a team of professionals. Consult your pediatrician and a speech-language pathologist.

25

How do auditory processing disorders affect classroom performance?

If a child has been diagnosed with an auditory processing disorder, it is likely that the instructor will observe the following behaviors in the classroom:

Difficulty following lengthy or complex instructions. This can be evident in any subject where there is a series of instructions to follow to understand and complete the task. Often these children will also have difficulty sequencing information in a logical order. For example, if there is a science experiment involving a series of steps that must be completed in sequence to ensure the success of the experiment, the child will tend to complete step 1, then skip to step 3, and then go back to step 2. This is minimized if the instructions can be written or depicted with pictures or graphics.

Decreased attention span. A frequent complaint of many teachers is that the child is "looking around the room when he should be paying attention." Often the lack of attention is a result of the inability to accurately process what the teacher said the first time. A natural tendency for most children is to observe what others are doing when they feel that they have missed something.

Distractibility in the presence of noise. Children with auditory processing disorders often have difficulty filtering out the background noises from important messages. As a result, everything floods into the system, and the child will have considerable difficulty deciphering the message.

Poor task completion. If the child does not process the instructions the first time, it is unlikely that he will successfully finish a project without having the instructions repeated.

Inappropriate or bizarre responses to instructor questions. If the information that the child hears is garbled nonsense, he will respond to what he thought he heard. For example, if the teacher asks, "What did you have for lunch today?" the child might respond, "My dog likes to eat hot dogs."

Parent Strategy

It may be helpful to the parent to know that instructors can make modifications in the classroom that will help the child process information. Here are some guidelines for teachers:

1. Seat the child in the front of the room in a location that will allow him to see you during a lesson. This will also aid in limiting the number of visual distractions. The more children seated between you and the child, the more opportunity the child will have to be easily distracted.

2. While you are at the board instructing, keep your face visible to the child whenever possible.

3. Always get the child's attention before asking a question or explaining information.

4. Eliminate any competing distractions, either visual or auditory. This includes not seating the child near a doorway or facing the window.

5. Simplify the instructions if the child does not get the information the first time. Do this by shortening the length of instructions, substituting less complex vocabulary words and concepts, and reducing the number of parts (that is, if you gave a two-part command, reduce it to one part). It may be helpful to break down

each task and write it down step by step for older children who are reading. Use visual diagrams to reinforce ideas for younger children.

6. Have the child rephrase what was said back to you to check for adequate processing. Exactness is not essential, but content of information is.

26

How do auditory processing disorders affect language skills?

We learn language through many channels, but the primary mode of learning is the auditory mode—listening to the language patterns of those around us as well as to ourselves. If the auditory channel is deficient in handling incoming information, this will affect not only the quality of receptive language that is developed and understood, but also the expressive use of that language. (Receptive language refers to the ability to understand what is spoken to us. Expressive language refers to what is expressed or spoken.) In the case of language abilities, an individual will be able to produce only what is readily understood. Thus, if the child has difficulty understanding and processing what is said to her, she will have equal difficulty in expressing herself.

This is exemplified in children who have poor oral language and discourse skills (conversational ability). During the years that I spent evaluating hundreds of school-aged children, a strong correlation emerged between the strength of auditory processing ability and expressive language skills. Often children who had difficulty organizing and understanding incoming information displayed equally poor ability in organizing expressive output. Discourse or conversation was often poorly sequenced and organized, limited in specific details and content, reduced in cohesiveness and coherence, and at times lacking in logic and appropriateness.

To oversimplify, if the information coming in lacks organization and sense to the child because of deficient processing of the message, what the child says in response to that input will reflect this. This lack of organization in oral language is sometimes reflected in written language as well. Our thoughts and ideas are the initiators of both the spoken and written word. Both oral and written language are expressive skills—one is verbal, the other graphic. If our thoughts and ideas are poorly organized, this will likely surface both in oral language and in writing.

Parent Strategy

If you suspect that your child has a language difficulty in addition to an auditory processing problem, seek the assistance of a speech-language pathologist for a complete evaluation. If an auditory processing problem is diagnosed, use the parent strategies outlined in questions 22 and 23. Depending upon the specific pattern exhibited, ask your speech-language pathologist for a home program that incorporates the development of age-appropriate language skills with auditory processing.

27

If after a formal diagnosis it is found that my child has an auditory processing deficit, will he outgrow it?

This is a common concern of many parents but difficult to answer. Often auditory processing abilities improve simply because of maturation; the neurological system gains maturity and skill out of experience and use. From my experience and observations of children who were diagnosed in elementary school and then followed through senior high school, auditory processing ability had improved but may not have achieved the same level as that of their peers.

It may be realistic to say that, although a parent can expect the child's abilities to improve, the underlying difficulty may still persist. It is therefore essential that a child be taught early how to use compensatory strategies to work around the problem (for example, use a tape recorder in class, write all information down, use organizational strategies), and to capitalize on the child's strengths and primary mode of learning, particularly if this mode is visual. This may mean presenting information consistently in a visual mode to augment the auditory information. Finally, simply because a child has been diagnosed as having these difficulties does not imply poor intellectual ability. Auditory processing disorders are nondiscriminatory: they affect all ages, races, genders, and levels of intelligence.

Parent Strategy

In addition to following the above recommendations, it is essential to pinpoint your child's strengths and develop these to the fullest. It is easy to overlook the more subtle inherent talents a child possesses when obvious problems are displayed so readily. Many of the same children who have a significant auditory processing deficit will be our architects, artists, scientists, and teachers of tomorrow. It may just take harder work and an alternative route to get there.

28

Sometimes my child will answer my questions or directives with an unusual response. It is very inappropriate and appears as if she is responding to a completely different question. What is going on?

This again relates to how much information actually got to the cortical level of the brain for processing. It could be that your child processed just bits and pieces of the message, with the rest being lost in transition from the ears through the auditory pathways to the brain. If this was the case, the child's response will reflect what she thought she heard. If your child heard garbled nonsense, her response will be nonsensical. For example, if you ask, "Where are your shoes?" and she responds, "I'm walking to school," I would question what information she is processing.

On the other hand, if you do not suspect an auditory processing difficulty, your child could very well have a pragmatics disorder. This is generally associated with the lack of socially appropriate usage of language in different communication situations. For example, if your child sees a boy fall off his bike and badly scrape a knee, and she teases him about why he is crying until his indignant mother arrives, your child has probably not learned the fine art of pragmatics: how to receive and transmit information for useful purposes in everyday situations. The social context in which the communication occurs is critical. If the child is able to read that social context appropriately and therefore use socially acceptable language for that situation, then pragmatics is not a concern.

Parent Strategy

Contact a speech-language pathologist and audiologist for a complete evaluation. It is essential first to rule out any hearing loss, followed by any auditory processing deficit. If both are absent, and the diagnosis indicates a language-related deficit in pragmatics, request a home program from the diagnosing speech-language pathologist to work on these skills. Follow parent recommendations for altering your behavior when speaking to your child (shorter, less complex instructions; visual cues; and so on).

29

If I ask my child to do something, it is as if he cannot remember from one moment to the next. However, he can remember what happened last year during vacation. What is this?

This is the difference between long-term and short-term auditory memory. In this example, the child has better long-term memory than short-term. Auditory processing of information is closely linked to memory. Short-term memory refers to immediate recall of information. Long-term refers to what occurred at some point in the past.

Short-term auditory memory problems affect not only the ability to immediately repeat or recall information, but the child's ability to remember and execute spoken directions with accuracy. Children with these deficits also display difficulty recalling the details and sequence of the instructions. As a result, these children may leave out or substitute words, phrases, or other essential details and become completely confused. For example, if you told your child, "Drink your milk, feed the cat, and water the lawn," he may give the cat water, drink his milk, and forget the rest.

Often there is a fine line between inefficient auditory processing and poor auditory memory. Some children may have adequate processing skills but deficient short-term auditory memory. However, others may have adequate auditory memory but poor processing skills. Some children have equally poor skills in both. It is essential to bear in mind that processing and memory are intertwined, and that a deficiency in one area can influence the other.

Parent Strategy

There are certain strategies that parents can use to aid in the recall of information. First, parents must teach their children three essential concepts: selecting, remembering, and reviewing (Strichart and Mangrum 1993, 8–12).

1. *Selecting:* We are exposed to large quantities of information each day. It is essential to decide what the key elements are in a message that are worthy of remembering.

2. *Remembering:* Select a technique that will facilitate in recalling the information. The technique selected depends on what is most appropriate for that situation at a given time.

   - *Visualizing:* At times it may be helpful to have your child picture in his mind what he is attempting to remember. For example, if trying to remember the directions on how to get somewhere, the child could visualize the road and picture himself bicycling or walking by each landmark on the way to the final destination.

   - *Associating:* With this technique, an item is related or connected to another item as a means of triggering memory. For example, if the child were required to remember a list of items such as dog, cat, shirt, mouse, and shoe, then teach the child to pair all the animals together in one set, and the clothing in another. This will reduce the items to two sets with fewer members in each group, making it easier to remember.

     A similar technique is referred to as "chunking." If a child is attempting to remember a phone number, the numbers can be repeated back in such a way as to "chunk" the numbers together. For example, the phone number 278-4800 can be rehearsed verbally as 27-84-800 or 278-48-00. Breaking the unit down into subgroups will facilitate memory.

- *Applying:* Providing the hands-on experience of applying an event or task to real life makes memorization easier. For example, the mathematical concept of multiplication will be remembered more easily if the child uses it to calculate how many oranges in four bags, rather than trying to learn it by rote memorization.

- *Repeating:* Have your child say, look at, and/or write the information repeatedly. Using all three methods simultaneously will facilitate retention most efficiently.

- *Mnemonic devices:* Acronyms, abbreviations, rhymes, and other devices are often used to aid in the improvement of memory. For example, if you wanted to remember to cut your hair, eat lunch with a friend, and go the library, you could create an acronym such as "CEL" to represent cut, eat, and library. Many mnemonic devices are rather complicated for most children to use, however, and are not highly recommended for younger children.

3. *Reviewing:* This stage enables the individual to remember information over a period of time. Techniques are simply not enough, because information that is not used is quickly lost from memory. There are three primary things the child must do to remember over a period of time:

- Reread information to be remembered.

- Recite information—say aloud the information to be remembered immediately after rereading it. This is also called verbal rehearsal.

- Rewrite information using key words, phrases, and abbreviations.

Repeat the above three steps again and again to remember over a period of time. The longer the information is to be remembered, the longer the child should cycle through these three steps.

30

How can parents help their children develop good listening and auditory processing skills?

Good listening skills start with good role models. Don't expect your child to develop either good listening or auditory processing skills without practice. Sitting in front of the television or Nintendo every night will certainly develop your child's visual skills or eye-hand co-ordination, but development and expansion of listening ability is questionable.

When a child is in the classroom, there is not going to be a command performance by the instructor if the child doesn't catch the information the first time. And if a child has not started to develop appropriate listening skills by the time she reaches school age, it may produce considerable problems academically.

If you expect your child to listen in the classroom, teach her to listen at home first. This starts with activities that promote listening in an active rather than a passive role, and continually challenge the auditory system to handle more complexity.

Parent Strategy

First realize that in any skill, including listening, "practice makes perfect." We can all become better at anything by practicing the skill. When a child watches television, she will certainly use both the visual and auditory modes (listening and watching). However, television does not require us to listen intently to the subject matter, because all spoken material is backed up with the actions on the screen. Thus, if we miss something, it doesn't take us long to figure out the missing link if we continue to watch the activity played out on the television. We are taught to rely more on the visual input than on key information obtainable by listening.

Also, watching a television does not present any opportunities for the type of interaction needed for listening or processing to be practiced. For listening and processing to occur, there must be an interplay of information or communication between two or more individuals that utilizes both the roles of speaker and listener within conversation. It is essential that you use whatever opportunities are available in the conversational setting to talk and listen to your child. A child will become a better listener and speaker as an adult if she has strong models to imitate when younger.

One tool I recommend to parents that cannot be stressed enough is books. Not only do books facilitate listening and processing, but they also open the doors to improved language, reading, writing, and memory. And without these prerequisites, it will be difficult for your child to be successful, whether she chooses to be a physician, an artist, or a mechanic. Read aloud to your child each evening. Ask her questions about what was read: the characters, the events, the problems, the solutions. If your child cannot get the gist of the story after reading through in its entirety and then asking questions, stop after each page or even each paragraph to determine how much information your child is really processing.

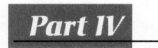

Part IV

Language Issues

Language defined: Language is a complex set of rules and symbols used to relay information between individuals, whether that information is expressed (spoken or signed) or understood.

31

What can I use as a general guide to determine whether my child is developing language adequately during the first few critical years?

The development of language skills can be broken down into receptive language and expressive language. As mentioned in Part III, receptive language refers to the ability to understand what is spoken to us. Expressive language refers to what we express or speak.

During the first twelve months of life, receptive language skills are intricately interwoven with cognitive skills: the child's knowledge of the world. For language skills to emerge, children must develop certain cognitive prerequisites. This cognitive awareness or knowledge comes from the interaction between the child and the objects and persons in his environment. For that reason, in Language Development Guide A after question 40, some receptive skills are interchangeable with cognitive behaviors.

Developmentally, a child will understand a concept long before he is able to express it. Therefore, if you wish your child to say the word "ball," you must first get him to understand what it is by exposing him to the object via play, talking, and saying the word numerous times in different contexts. Only when your child has developed sufficient understanding of the concept will he be ready to use the word expressively, and this will also be when the child's articulatory or speech patterns develop to the point where he is ready to place the tongue in at least the approximately correct posture for the production of sounds.

Parent Strategy

When utilizing Language Development Guide A, once again keep in mind that your child will understand a concept receptively before using it expressively. Also, remember that developmental milestone charts are only guides, and that simply because a child says his first words at fourteen months rather than eleven or twelve months does not constitute a language difficulty or disorder. Finally, the emphasis here will be on the first five years of life, which are the most critical years for language development and will provide the solid basis for future growth. The quantity as well as the quality of time you spend with your child during these years is the prerequisite to successful learning in the future. See Language Development Guides A and B after question 40.

32

If there is a difficulty in acquiring language skills, what areas are typically affected?

When a child speaks her first words, the underlying language processes involve the following parameters: semantics, syntax, morphology, and pragmatics. Semantics refers to word meaning, content, or vocabulary used. Syntax refers to word order within the sentence. Morphology pertains to the smallest meaningful unit of speech and includes such items as plurals (book vs. books), verb tenses (jumped, jumping, will jump), articles (the, a, an), and prepositions. Pragmatics refers to how appropriately the child uses the language she learns. For example, socially inappropriate responses to questions would be considered a pragmatic difficulty. Here is one example:

Parent: What do you like to eat at McDonald's?

Child: A hamburger, fries. . . I don't go to McDonald's for breakfast.

Parent: Why not?

Child: Well, you know I used to sleep in New Jersey. I used to go to a motel and I don't eat breakfast. You know that one sandwich? It was in Pennsylvania.

Parent Strategy

How would a parent know if her child has a language difficulty? Using Language Development Guides A and B after question 40, look at several factors: Did your child develop most skills within a reasonable time frame (age of first words, putting two words together, etc.)? Where is your child's vocabulary now, either receptively or expressively, particularly after age one? How are your child's listening skills, particularly in view of her current age level? Are there any factors present from birth that will influence language (e.g., cerebral palsy, hearing loss)? Finally, realize that many children go through stages of language development where errors are a part of the process. Simply because a child is saying "I comed home" for "I came home" is not reason enough to warrant alarm. Also, when children learn new vocabulary it is not uncommon for them to "overgeneralize" this label to everything. Thus, the word "daddy" may be given to every male the child sees, or every dog the child sees has the same name as her family pet. This is a normal process. However, if you suspect that your child is not learning language and achieving key milestones within a reasonable age range (see Language Development Guides A and B after question 40), consult a speech-language pathologist (SLP).

33

How can parents help develop their child's vocabulary?

A child's expressive vocabulary begins with the appearance of the first word around the age of ten to fourteen months. However, as mentioned earlier, a child's receptive knowledge or comprehension of that word starts long before that. The production of the first word is dependent on the following factors (Dale 1976, 7): evidence of understanding what the word is (receptive knowledge), consistent and spontaneous use of the word (not just imitation of the adult), and the word's being one that is part of the adult's language (e.g., an adult would not use "waba" for "cat"). First words are almost always one or two syllables, are usually a consonant-vowel combination, and usually begin with consonants that are visible when spoken by others ("p," "b," "d," "t," "m," and "n"). Thus, "mama" and "papa" are common first words. First words can also typically be approximations of the adult word such as "gog" for "dog."

Parent Strategy

The following are suggested guidelines when aiding in the growth of your child's vocabulary:

1. *Reception precedes expression:* People learn language and vocabulary by listening to and watching the world around them. When we constantly stimulate the child's auditory, visual, and tactile systems (talk to him, read aloud, provide experiences to touch and feel his surroundings), a child will acquire knowledge of the world. Furthermore, the child requires constant exposure to his environment through listening, seeing, and touching to develop a complex system of communicating we know as language. Therefore, it is essential that the child's experiences precede actual receptive knowledge. It is only when the child has acquired an adequate understanding of a concept that he is able to express it. Thus, it is common that a child will point to or identify a picture or object before expression of that picture or object occurs.

2. *Types of words acquired:* From the research completed in the area of language, general nouns or names of persons, places, or things are the most common vocabulary items to be developed first (e.g., "ball," "doggie"). Specific names of persons such as "mommy" or pets or the specific pet name such as "Polly" are also common (Dale 1976, 8–9).

   Action words are the next most frequently occurring words in a child's vocabulary and can include words such as "bye-bye," "give," and "up." Modifiers (e.g., "red," "dirty") and personal-social words (e.g., "yes," "no," "please") are less common.

   Finally, a child will be likely to acquire a word in his vocabulary if it is something that he can act upon. For example, it would be more likely that the child would learn the words "socks" or "hat" rather than "pants" or "diaper" simply because the child can act upon the previous items—he can find them, take them off, or put them on. Also, change is important: objects that change and move themselves (cars, clocks, animals, etc.) are likely to be named. But in terms of what he learns to name first, change induced by the child will be the most influential (Dale 1976, 9).

3. *Objects versus pictures:* Real objects will always be superior in teaching new vocabulary over pictures in a book. Let the child feel the item when the word is spoken for the object. Since most of the first words are nouns, many of these items are found around the home and are specific to your child's interests and experiences. When developing knowledge of action words, acting these out with bodily gestures and facial expressions while playing would be helpful. If you choose books to teach vocabulary, select books that have color photographs (preferable over drawings), are colorful, and represent words that are relevant to your child's world.

4. *Developmental level:* Knowing your child's developmental level is essential when teaching vocabulary, particularly if you decide to use picture books to strengthen vocabulary. For example, you would not select a book containing three-syllable words if you had a ten-month-old who is just starting to develop an interest in looking at books. Choose books that have monosyllabic (one-syllable) words beginning with sounds that are easily visible ("p,"

"b," "m," "n," "t," "d"), and that your child can relate to or that contain the most meaning for him. However, books can never replace the interaction the child can get in the early years with the parent, real objects, and experiences in the environment. Talk to your child about what you see around you. This not only provides a language model to the child, but develops those auditory and listening skills that are so essential to future language growth and academic success.

Prior to the age of nine or ten months, focus vocabulary enrichment on activities that involve direct activity with both you, the parent, and toys the child can act upon and influence. The first nine months will be a period where the child learns by being an active listener, watcher, and toucher of the world around him. When he has acquired enough exposure to that world through the senses (auditory, visual, and tactile), it is only then that he will begin expressing what he experiences in that world. Use the first half of Language Development Guide A after question 40 as a tool to aid you in toy selection and activities, and talk to your child from birth onward. It is never too early to start on developing language. Finally, use the following techniques to aid in the facilitation of language:

1. *Self-talk:* Use simple, clear, speech to describe what you are doing, how you are doing it, and so on. Keep the speech rate slow.

2. *Parallel talk:* While your child is engaged in activity, talk about what he is doing. Do not force your child to talk, but rather encourage him to speak about what he is doing.

3. *Imitation:* Encourage your child to imitate your words or phrases when he wishes to, rather than forcing it. Reinforce any imitative efforts.

4. *Modeling:* Whenever your child says something, try to elaborate on what was said. For example, if he said "kitty nice," you could follow that with, "Yes, the kitty is soft and gray."

5. *Expansion:* If your child makes either an incomplete or grammatically incorrect statement, use the child's own words to elaborate to make the statement complete. For example, if the

child said, "dog run," you could expand by saying, "Yes, the dog is running."

6. *Prompting:* If your child fails to respond to a question you ask, modify your question. For example, if you said, "Where did you go?" you could restate this as "You went where?"

As a last suggestion, try not to anticipate your child's needs by making language unnecessary. If you know what your child wants, don't immediately get it for him without at least some vocalization, even if it is unintelligible. Simply pointing to what is wanted is not helpful in aiding vocabulary development. After the child has made a vocalization or attempt to respond (gesturing along with the vocalization is fine), then name the desired object, encourage but don't demand that he attempt to imitate you, then give him the object or toy. Remember to talk constantly about your environment—what is happening or exists around you. Try to avoid approaching language by walking around and asking repeatedly, "What is this, what is that?" This is acceptable when used in conjunction with other methods, but not by itself.

Most children acquire at least fifty words expressively before they are able to put two or more words together. Every child is different, so allow your child to go at his own pace, and provide plenty of meaningful experiences and opportunities for him to explore and learn about the world around him.

34

I am ready to purchase the first books for my child. What advice would be helpful in book selection when the goal is language development?

Remember these general rules:

- Know the developmental level of your child.
- Experiences precede receptive knowledge.
- Receptive language precedes expressive language.
- Nouns and action words develop before other words.

- Choose books with photographs or realistic drawings.
- Choose color versus black and white illustrations.
- Choose books that show items the child can act upon or influence.
- Stick to monosyllabic words (no more than two syllables for first books).
- Find words beginning with easily visible sounds ("p," "t," "m," "b," "d," "n").

Parent Strategy

Ask yourself the following questions whenever you are selecting a first book for your child:

Are the pictures realistic? Color photographs are great, but there are many books that have realistic drawings. Use your own judgment and knowledge of what appeals to your child. The more realistic, the better.

Are there too many pictures on each page? Your goal is to expose your child to the pictures, not visually distract her. One or two pictures per page in a concept book is plenty for the child who is looking at books for the first time.

Are the pictures and vocabulary in the book developmentally appropriate for your child? Are they simple and to the point? Some words suitable for the toddler to learn would be unsuitable for the three- or four-year-old, and vice versa. If your focus is to teach the concept of "truck" to the child who is looking at books for the first time, don't confuse the issue by selecting books that show a picture of a truck with the printed word "vehicle" underneath. I would question picture books that have any printed material under the picture if this is your child's first book, because the book is intended to aid your child in getting familiar with books, not to read printed material that she won't be ready for until a few years later. If you wish to expose the infant to printed material with pictures, think developmentally: familiarization with the individual letters (along with colorful pictures) would be more practical and realistic, but realize that reading is not your goal at this point.

What about your child's fine motor and grasping skills? Is she able to turn pages or hold the book in her lap? Children develop an interest in books long before their motor skills catch up to enable them to turn the pages independently, so be aware of this. At approximately six months of age, the palm and fingers are used to grossly grasp objects. A precise pincer grasp with thumb opposition (a more mature pattern) won't develop until later (usually around one year). Therefore, choose books that are easy for your child to handle given her limited fine motor skills during the first year. Books with heavy cardboard pages are convenient, particularly when everything goes into the child's mouth or will get torn easily. Also, books that are about 5" x 7" or 3" x 5" in size are more realistic for children this age rather than large, bulky books, or very tiny books. Simply because the child is miniature in size doesn't mean the books have to be.

What about the child's attention span and visual skills? Does she focus on the pictures in a book or show no interest? Consult Language Development Guides A and B after question 40. Infants are able to look at pictures up to approximately one minute at about eight to nine months. It isn't until about age ten to fourteen months that the child starts to really enjoy looking at books; most children assist in turning pages at approximately fourteen to eighteen months.

Are the pictures and vocabulary depicted useful based upon your child's experiences? I cringe whenever I see a child's first picture book in the bookstores with the standard ten pictures, and the same redundant theme: car, mom, bed, dog, ball, and so on. This is adequate if these items are the most meaningful to your child, but chances are they are not. Only you can be the best judge of what interests your child. Therefore, I recommend that you develop your own "first books" that are meaningful for your child by doing the following:

1. Take color photographs of items that your child loves. More than likely these will be animals, people, or things that the child can influence or act upon, or that have the capability of changing themselves after the child has acted upon them, such as a wind-up toy. This may include significant family members (not just mom and dad), family pets, favorite toys, clothing (socks and shoes would be easier for the child to act upon than a diaper or a

sweater, so include these as part of her first picture book). When taking the photographs, keep background distractions to a minimum. For example, if you photograph a favorite toy sitting on the television, are you teaching the concept of the toy or the television?

2. Try to select words that meet the criteria in item 1, but are monosyllabic (one syllable). Bisyllabic words are not forbidden but may be more difficult for your child to express when she is ready to do so. Remember that words containing the most visible speech sounds ("b," "p," "t," "d," "m," "n") will be easier, particularly if they begin with this sound. However, if the word has a lot of meaning to your child and doesn't begin with one of these sounds, include it in her book.

3. Take the color photographs and paste one photograph per page, preferably on heavier construction paper or posterboard. You may wish to cut the paper down into more manageable sizes for ease of handling (e.g., 6" x 6" pieces). Punch holes in the side of the paper and place the sheets into a notebook or binder. You may also wish to cover the pages with plastic to protect the photos, and to protect your child's fingers from picking up any photographic chemicals if wet.

4. Select about ten to fifteen words to begin with. Initially, point to and name the picture or the object. Simply have the child watch and listen as you go through the pictures. Eventually, when your child has been exposed to the pictures over a period of time, you can then progress to asking the child "Where is the _____?" and having the child point to it. When the child consistently understands a concept, this will open the way to expressing it.

5. You may question why it would be important to make a book out of your child's favorite items in the home when it would be just as easy to allow the child to play with the real thing. Real objects are necessary to developing language, but placing these in a book format will ready the child to move into the next stages of development. Books teach the child visual discrimination, development of attention span, and most important, listening. The child will rely more and more on these skills as she matures.

Finally, when I see all of the first picture books in the stores neatly sorted by classification and category (furniture, clothing, food, colors, etc.), I have to wonder if the commonly held belief is that this is how the first vocabulary is developed. It is certainly a very well organized way to try to define language, but it is too narrowly focused. If you wish to teach your child these concepts, try to select books that introduce them within a story format. At least in this way the vocabulary is used in a meaningful context rather than in a sequence of unrelated and isolated pictures. Review again what is useful and meaningful to your child and her interests. Teach what is important in her understanding of her world, not how to categorize a word into a larger group. If you feel the urge to have the vocabulary neatly organized by category books, then make your own book that is specific to your child's world and experiences by following the suggestions above.

In conclusion, never forget the importance of developmental progression of language concepts. So many books include pictures of nouns alone; of nouns functioning as objects of verbs and prepositions; of colors, shapes, and opposites—all introduced in the same book. Nouns are certainly viable for a first picture book, but the latter concepts are suitable for a much older population (see Language Developmental Guides A and B after question 40).

35

I try to read a book to my child at bedtime each evening. What are some suggestions to improve language skills during story time?

As children mature beyond the first year, their interest in books and stories develops dramatically. Because many parents use story time in the evening to spend time with their children, this is also an excellent opportunity to develop language skills in the area of comprehension, oral language, vocabulary, and memory for information.

Parent Strategy

The essential basic element to any story is the vocabulary being used. If you are using a picture book, does your child know the names of the items in the picture? It would be difficult at best for a child to retell his own version of the story without knowing the vocabulary.

For children who are not yet readers, I highly recommend using a wordless picture book to develop these skills. First, go through the book with your child and talk about the pictures. Talk about the names of the objects seen in the pictures, the actions taking place, and the feelings and emotions depicted on the characters' faces. Then start at the beginning of the book and make up your own story about what is happening, being sure to include all essential details, actions, and characters, with a clear beginning, middle, and end to the story.

For the older child, in addition to the above, after you have told a story using the pictures (with your child listening only), go through the story page by page and ask questions about what is happening. Check for comprehension and memory by asking questions such as:

"What were the names of the characters in the story?"

"What problem did the characters encounter?"

"How did the characters feel about certain events?"

"How was the problem solved?"

"How would you solve the problem if you were one of the characters?"

"Was there a lesson or moral to the story?"

These questions are more suited for the child who has been looking at books for a few years, and they assume good expressive usage of language.

If your child has difficulty remembering information, it may be helpful to break the story down. After reading the story once in its entirety, go through the book and read the story page by page. After you have completed one page, ask questions about what was read. If your child still has difficulty, break it down even further, by paragraph. Read a paragraph, then ask questions about it. Try not to pressure your child. Sharing a story should be a pleasant time for you and your child, and if it turns out to be a drill exercise, go back to just telling the story with your child actively listening.

If your child is six or older, have him go through the book and make up his own story. Make sure he is not just describing isolated events pictured on each page. The story must be cohesive and flow together in a logical sequence. When a child orally tells a story either from a picture book or from memory, the story will generally contain a narrative core. Most children are able to establish a narrative core by the time they reach early elementary school. The narrative core should contain the following:

a clear beginning, middle, and end to the story line

the setting in which the story took place

the characters involved in the story

a problem or dilemma in the story

an attempt or plan of action to resolve the problem

the consequences of the attempted action

the overall theme or moral to the story

When the older child has developed written language skills, oral language can be used to aid written language. If a child is having difficulty writing his own story, for example, it may be helpful to have the child say out loud what he wants to say before writing it down. The same is true for oral language. If the child is having difficulty organizing orally what he wishes to say, writing the information down first will be helpful.

Another useful exercise for older children is to select several vocabulary words from the story. Then have the child rewrite the story using synonyms (words having the same meaning) instead of the original vocabulary words. Also, talk about word opposites. Randomly select words from the story and determine their opposite meaning ("strong" means "not _____"). Do not hesitate to teach your child to use a dictionary or thesaurus rather than get the answers from you.

Finally, if your child has spelling words to learn each week, use this as an opportunity to develop vocabulary and storytelling skills. First have him make up a sentence (orally) using the spelling word. Then have him write the sentence down. Follow this by having your child make up a short story using all the spelling words, in writing or orally.

36

What activities are most helpful to the parent of a new baby to facilitate language growth?

When a newborn or child learns language, there is first an assumption that all the senses are intact (hearing, vision, touch, etc.). If this is not the case, there are now early intervention programs available to assist parents as early as the first month of life to support them in whatever area needs specialized attention.

The development of language first begins with getting the infant to tune her senses in to her immediate surroundings. This includes fine-tuning the visual, auditory, and tactile skills. An infant's auditory system will first respond to gross sounds during the first month of life; it will then respond to the human voice by the second month. Gradually the infant learns to focus more intently on the human voice for longer periods of time, and usually by approximately age two to three months the infant will search with the eyes when a sound is heard.

It is also during this time (two to three months of age) that the infant will watch the speaker's mouth and eyes, an important milestone and prerequisite for communication. Gradually between the ages of three and five months, the infant will localize sound with the eyes (eyes shifting to the source of sound). By the time the infant reaches the age of six months, she will be able to localize tactile stimulation by touching the same spot or searching for the object that touched the body. Thus, it is quite clear that during the first six months of life, the auditory, tactile, and visual systems are preparing and developing the capability to handle a more complex method of communicating.

Parent Strategy

So how does the parent stimulate these sensory systems in the infant? To develop the infant's sense of hearing, it is essential that parents talk to their child from the moment of birth. Simply because an infant has not developed the capability of understanding words does not mean that she is incapable of communicating. During the first months of life, infants will communicate without words by watching your face when you speak, cooing or crying when they are either pleased or unhappy, listening intently to different sounds and voices around them, and placing everything in the mouth.

Each of these senses (hearing, sight, and touch) provides the feedback and information the infant needs to learn more about her environment. It is essential that as a parent you are there to provide that stimulation to develop those senses. If an infant is placed into a nonstimulating environment, either visually, auditorially, or tactilely, the end result on developing communication skills will be dramatically reduced.

Therefore, talk to your infant; repeat back any noises, cooing, or babbling that your child engages in. Sing songs, repeat nursery rhymes, and read simple poetry and stories, even if she isn't old enough to understand them. Make sure that your child can see your face when you speak to her, and provide her with a stimulating visual and tactile environment through toys, games, books, and experiences. And remember that infants will attain much of their knowledge of the world by placing whatever they can in the mouth, so select toys that are suitable for their age level.

Finally, refer to question 31. The sensory systems will always inherently be integrated with the ability to develop language, and the cognitive and receptive prerequisites are essential to a strong foundation.

37

How can I incorporate teaching language skills into hectic daily routines?

The most effective way to fit language learning activities into daily routines is to approach the interactions you have with your child as opportunities for learning. In this way, you are already using the existing and naturally occurring situations to expound on. The most essential thing to remember is that the learning situation should be natural and realistic, rather than contrived and artificial. All of the following suggestions assume that the child is speaking in sentences.

Parent Strategy

A parent can take advantage of a naturally occurring situation to develop language skills in each of the following areas:

Problem solving: Let us assume that you are driving down the highway and you see a man pulled over with a flat tire. Ask your child the following questions:

How could the man solve the problem of the flat tire?

If the man had no spare tire, what else could he do?

How do you think the tire became flat? What was the cause?

Why couldn't the man just inflate the tire again with air?

What could the man have done to avoid getting a flat tire?

By asking these types of questions, you engage your child in actively using language to solve problems, think ahead, and develop an association of cause and effect. Some research has found that many children and adolescents with behavioral problems simply have not developed these problem-solving skills or were not taught by their parents to solve problems. These types of questions can be used in any situation where there is a predicament to resolve or alternative choices to make.

Discourse and oral language: As children develop their expressive language skills, they become proficient at conversational language, which speech-language pathologists refer to as discourse. Discourse involves many different abilities and assumes that the child's oral language will contain the following:

- appropriate word order, sentence length, and grammar
- appropriate vocabulary usage
- enough information so that the listener is not confused
- accurate information
- completion of a thought or topic before progressing to a new idea
- socially appropriate usage in a given environment or situation, such as not swearing or using slang

■ adequate verbal organization with limited use of revisions, delays, or hesitations

Like any skill, whether it be sports, playing music, or drawing, expressive language proficiency improves with practice and repetition. Not only will practice with oral language tasks improve the child's overall skill level, but his self-confidence in these situations will dramatically improve as well. Remember to use the techniques outlined in question 33 (modeling, expansion, etc.) when attempting to facilitate language growth.

With younger children (early elementary school and preschool), use wordless picture books to guide the child in making up his own stories out loud. Look for completeness, description of characters and activities, an organized and coherent sequence of events, and usage of appropriate vocabulary.

For the older child, encourage involvement in speech or debate teams, theatre, and public speaking classes. Although many of us dread public speaking situations, with practice the stress and discomfort levels will be reduced considerably.

Vocabulary: Start by encouraging your child to read and to love reading from an early age. Children who do the best academically are those who have strong reading skills and continue to expand on those skills by opening themselves to the world of books. A love of reading and books is taught by the parent and doesn't start when the child reaches school age. It starts in infancy, when your child is old enough to have an attention span long enough to look at you when you are speaking.

You and your child will never be too old to learn new vocabulary. The homework your child brings home each night is a prime opportunity to work on vocabulary. For example, when your child brings spelling words home each week, do you take the time to not only work on the spelling but to check on whether your child understands what they mean? Have your child tell you what the word means or use the word in a sentence either by writing it down or saying it out loud. Talk about synonymous word meanings (words that mean the same thing). If the word is "big," does your child know that it can also mean "huge," "large," and so on? Does your child know that the opposite of "big" is "small," "tiny," "little," and so on?

When your child has a reading assignment, does he understand the vocabulary being used? When you read stories to your child, can he decipher the meaning of the words in the story by the context in which they are used? Discuss the words in the stories you read to your child. Don't assume anything.

Listening and auditory processing: I cannot stress enough that television is no substitute for human communication. Certainly there are some excellent children's programs on the air, but these will never take the place of the roles we take on as listener and speaker when engaged in conversation.

If you want your child to develop good listening skills and carry them into the classroom, you have to provide the opportunity for this to happen. Watching television all weekend and every day after school will not help. In addition, if you are not taking the time each day to listen to your child, don't expect him to listen to you. Take the time to be with, talk to, and listen to your child. Your time with him will go much farther than any of the best programs on television.

Grammar and syntax: Should you be overly concerned if your child is using improper grammar? This really depends on the frequency of errors and how much they interfere with your child's communication attempts. For many children, particularly when they are below age six, grammatical errors are a part of the developmental process. For example, if your child is saying "goed" for "went" or "eated" for "ate," simply model the correct production rather than demanding perfect production. Simply say, "Yes, the boy ate the sandwich," or "Oh, you mean the boy ate the sandwich." If you believe that the problem is more than developmental, contact a speech-language pathologist. Language Development Guides A and B after question 40 may be of assistance in determining whether your child's grammatical problems are more than developmental.

38

What are the effects of patent eustachian (PE) tube placement on language development?

See question 17 for a more detailed explanation of middle ear infection, or otitis media, and how the PE tubes are put into place.

PE tube placement itself is not necessarily the culprit. The actual presence of the infection and fluid accumulation are more the issue, because their influence on speech and language skills can be detrimental, particularly during the critical years of infancy to age three. However, there are studies stipulating that "parents and teachers need not be overly concerned about the effects of OME [otitis media effusion, or secretory otitis media] on later language development" (Grievink et al. 1993, 1011). These authors were eager to point out that their own conclusions "should be taken with caution," and that "further study is needed to determine if there are circumstances in which OME is a decisive factor in bringing about language disorders" (Grievink et al. 1993, 1011).

Therefore, be aware that controversy exists about the effects of middle ear infections on language skills, but that there is still a strong case for possible detrimental effects on language, particularly in the formative years. The placement of tubes in the ears and the resultant influence on language and speech skills will vary depending on several factors: the frequency and severity of the middle ear infections, the duration of the infections, and the age at which they occur. For example, a child who has frequent and chronic ear infections at age three will be more at risk for developing language or speech problems than a seven-year-old who gets the infection with a head cold. The first three to five years are considered to be one of the more critical periods in which speech and language skills develop, so any prolonged interference with this process would deter normal development.

So should you be concerned about PE tube placement? My response is that you should be more concerned about how soon treatment is initiated, how severe the infections are, how long they endure, and how frequently your child gets them. All these factors can certainly play a role in determining whether PE tube placement is necessary, and how long the tubes stay in the ears.

Another question is just as important: what skills will be affected if frequent and chronic ear infections interfere with development? Primarily, articulation may be affected; see question 17. Because the speech that the child hears will be distorted, she will reproduce what she believes she heard. Language skills could be delayed in a number of different areas. For example, the child may be taking longer to say her first words or put two words together to make her first sentences.

Grammar could be delayed as well as expanding vocabulary. If the child is speaking in sentences, overall sentence length may be reduced with limited complexity.

Parent Strategy

It is essential to get medical attention for your child as soon as possible if you suspect that she is developing a middle ear infection. If your child has a history of frequent ear infections, monitor her development using Language Development Guides A and B after question 40. You may also wish to consult a speech-language pathologist to screen your child to identify any problem areas or to rule out any concerns you may have.

39

My child appears to have a good vocabulary and is quite verbal, but it is difficult to follow what he is saying because he rambles and no thoughts are tied together. As a result, nothing appears to make sense. Does he have a problem?

This description is typical of children with discourse problems. Discourse refers to the child's ability to organize spoken language so that the listener understands what is being said. Often children with discourse problems are unable to provide enough information to the listener and are very vague and nondescriptive in their efforts to communicate. For example:

Parent: Are you going outside?

Child: No, I can stay inside with Jack. Yeah, OK . . . I'll stay inside with Jack. I'll do some work inside. Jack, Jack is gonna stay inside. Jill will go outside. Is she gone . . . Yeah . . . I can stay inside with Jack and color. Jill's gonna go out.

In the above example, the child simply rambles with no organization or clarity. In the example below, the child is unable to provide enough information:

Parent: Tell me about school.

Child: Fun.

Parent: What did you do at school?

Child: Stuff . . . some things.

Parent: What kinds of things?

Child: Them one things . . . you know.

In addition, topic maintenance (following a thought through from beginning to end) may be limited, with the obvious result being thoughts that jump from one item to the next with no cohesiveness. The child may also respond inappropriately to the communicative situation with unusual or weird responses, or display a speech style that is situationally inappropriate. Finally, these organizational deficits may come out in the form of constantly revising what is said, pausing or delaying the response, and using numerous fillers (e.g., "um," "uh") before or within a speech attempt.

Parent Strategy

Consult a speech-language pathologist to determine whether your child has a language disorder if you observe these behaviors. Correlative studies have shown that children who have poor oral discourse often have equally poor auditory processing ability. Thus, if a child has difficulty organizing and making sense of incoming information that he listens to (auditory processing), the output/spoken language will reflect those limitations. It will also be poorly organized and limited in cohesiveness. Request that your child also be tested for any auditory processing difficulty.

40

My oldest child said her first words and sentences at an early age, but my second child seems to be taking his time. Should I be concerned?

This depends on what "taking his time" means. If your second child is thirteen months old and hasn't said his first word, and your firstborn said her first word by eleven months, try not to make comparisons. Consult Language Development Guides A and B after question 40 and determine whether it really is a problem or if you have the expectation that your second child will be identical to your first. Most children learn language at their own pace within a time frame that is reasonable developmentally. Try not to make the assumption that all siblings will be the same developmentally, because they won't be—particularly boys versus girls. Girls tend to excel developmentally at an early age with language, and boys as a rule spend many years catching up to their female counterparts.

It is quite normal for older children to develop language skills at an earlier age than their younger siblings. As to why this happens, it could be any number of things. Some theorize that anxious parents the first time around are overzealous in their efforts to have the first baby not only excel, but surpass all existing developmental charts and predictions. Then when the second child arrives, they are more realistic about their expectations. Another belief is that if there is an older sibling around (particularly a verbal one), it is quite easy to allow the verbal sibling to do all the work. Also, there may well be fewer opportunities for the younger child to try out his communication skills if the older child monopolizes the conversation. Remember that developmental readiness is the key.

Parent Strategy

Try not to be overly concerned about differences among siblings when attaining speech and language milestones, unless you observe a behavior in your child that you feel is inappropriate on the basis of his current age level. Always consult a speech-language pathologist if you have concerns about delayed speech or language.

Language Development Guide A: The Growth of Receptive Language in Children from Birth to Five Years

Adapted from the SKI-HI Language Development Scale and from the American Speech and Hearing Association's pamphlet "How Does Your Child Hear and Talk?" Portions on grammatical development are adapted from an unpublished paper by Clara Jacobs and Carol Peterson, "A Developmental Scale of Syntactic Structures," Northwestern University, 1967.

This guide outlines the major developments in vocabulary, grammar, sentence length, and knowledge of basic concepts that occur in childrens' *receptive* language (understanding and comprehension) during the first five years of life.

Items in italics are cognitive prerequisites for language: behaviors that are viewed as necessary precursors to language.

Birth to two months

- is quieted by hearing a familiar voice or being picked up
- shows interest in watching the immediate environment
- reacts pleasurably when anticipating or expecting an event (e.g., mealtime)
- reacts to speaker by appearing to listen when the speaker is in close proximity
- responds with a startle to loud or unexpected sounds or noises
- ceases activity when hears sound or noise
- attends to other voices
- exhibits emerging auditory tracking/localizing behaviors (e.g., motions of body, blinks, or facial expressions indicate that sound was detected; moves head to source of sound)

Two to four months

- watches speaker's lips, mouth, and face during speech
- recognizes the sounds that precede an event such as being fed or picked up
- associates mother with certain noises or activities
- is aware of immediate environment, particularly certain sights and sounds
- is sensitive to unfamiliar situations or strange surroundings
- is usually made distraught by angry voices or facial expressions
- ceases crying or fussing if hears spoken words
- reacts to speech by searching and localizing speaker with eyes

- visually tracks objects (e.g., follows an object with the eyes either horizontally, vertically, or randomly)

Four to six months

- sometimes turns or looks up when name is called
- distinguishes between strangers and familiar persons
- begins to notice toys that make sounds
- responds to changes in another's tone of voice
- responds to "no" at least half of the time by withdrawing or ceasing activity
- begins to recognize words like "mama," "dada"
- looks around for the source of new sounds (doorbell, vacuum, etc.)
- exhibits awareness of emerging signs of object permanence (e.g., if toy is totally or partially hidden, child will search for it or notice its disappearance: this behavior can emerge at up to ten or eleven months)

Six to eight months

- recognizes words that are easily associated with a physical gesture, such as "hi," by responding with appropriate gesture
- begins to recognize the names of some common objects when heard
- begins to attend to music or song
- begins to recognize family members' names when spoken, even if person referred to is not present
- consistently ceases activity when own name is called

Eight to ten months

- follows some simple verbal directions (e.g., "wave bye-bye")
- generally gives toys or objects to parent when asked
- reacts to "no" consistently by ceasing activity
- sustains attention up to one minute when looking at pictures being named
- usually attends to speech in the presence of outside distractions

- obtains enjoyment from listening to new words
- develops awareness of cause and effect (e.g., looks at wind-up toy closely to investigate how it operates)

Ten to twelve months

- has increased attention span and response to speech over greater lengths of time
- more consistently follows simple commands and understands simple questions such as "roll the ball" or "where is your shoe?"
- responds with appropriate verbal response to requests to indicate comprehension of task (e.g., "say daddy" and child says "dada")
- reacts to music by moving hands or body in rhythm or time
- demonstrates means-to-end behaviors: uses a stick or other tool to reach a toy
- responds with appropriate gesture to verbal requests, demonstrating comprehension of task (e.g., "where's the ball?" and child points to it)

Twelve to fourteen months

- maintains interest in pictures named for up to two minutes
- after parental request, consistently gives toy to parent
- understands at least one familiar body part when named
- appears to understand the feelings and emotions of the speaker
- expands understanding of vocabulary with new words each week
- follows simple one-step instructions such as "get your ball"
- follows through on simple actions to pictures such as "kiss the baby"

Fourteen to sixteen months

- understands the names of many objects; points to or looks at object when named
- understands at least two familiar body parts when named
- understands simple verbal requests by following through with appropriate action (e.g., gets a favorite toy from another room)

- looks at and points to pictures when asked questions like "where is the dog?"
- demonstrates understanding of separation when parent is not physically present

Sixteen to eighteen months

- finds pleasure in listening to simple rhymes and songs
- follows through when given two directions using one object either consecutively or not (e.g., "Get your hat. Put the hat on.")
- correctly identifies or points to two or more from a group of at least four objects
- begins to associate words with the categories in which they belong (e.g., food, toys)
- finds enjoyment in looking at books, and turns pages independently

Eighteen to twenty months

- begins to understand possessive grammatical forms such as "mine"
- generalizes knowledge of at least three to four body parts on a doll or in a picture by pointing to them when named
- makes a distinction between personal pronouns such as "her," "him," "he," "she," "me," etc.
- responds appropriately to action words or phrases such as "hit ball"
- in the home, develops a knowledge of where common objects can be located (e.g., spoon in the kitchen)
- develops awareness of different colors

Twenty to twenty-two months

- responds to a series of up to two or three related commands (e.g., "Get the cat, pet the cat, give the cat to me.")
- expands comprehension of new vocabulary words daily
- enjoys listening to simple stories from books
- identifies five to six familiar body parts on a doll

- understands and identifies most common objects when named, either with real objects or in pictures
- identifies at least four items of clothing on self when named

Twenty-two to twenty-four months

- responds to a series of at least four related commands (e.g., "Get the ball, throw the ball, put the ball down, give the ball to me.")
- matches at least two colors and some familiar objects
- upon request, picks out one item from a group of at least five
- demonstrates interest in commercials on television and radio
- begins to understand adjectives in phrases such as "hot food," "dirty clothes," etc.
- understands simple pronouns better (e.g., "my," "you," "he," "she")
- begins to listen to the underlying meanings of language, not just the words and sounds heard
- comprehends complex sentences better (e.g., "When we get home, we'll watch a movie.")

Twenty-four to twenty-eight months

- comprehends verb forms and actions by identifying the action correctly in pictures (e.g., "point to playing")
- begins to understand number concepts such as "one" or "more than one"
- distinguishes between "mine" and "yours"
- distinguishes between the concepts of "same" and "different"
- is aware of self and family members in photos
- understands some family name categories (e.g., mother, sister, brother, father)
- begins to understand simple prepositional forms, such as "in" or "on"
- can sort pictures into categories (e.g., toys in one group, food in another)
- understands size concepts such as "big," "little," etc., in a group of objects

- understands less identifiable parts of the body (e.g., eyebrow, elbow, chin)

Twenty-eight to thirty-two months

- has increased understanding of most common verbs and actions (e.g., "play," "walk," "run")
- has increased comprehension of adjectives and descriptors (e.g., "hot," "dry," "pretty")
- has increased comprehension of long and complex sentences
- understands the function of some objects when asked (e.g., "Show me what we cut with": child points to scissors or knife)
- uses color to match objects
- begins to display turntaking and sharing behaviors

Thirty-two to thirty-six months (three years)

- responds appropriately to a three-part instruction when spoken within one sentence
- expands knowledge of prepositions and location words (such as "under," "over," etc.)
- indicates understanding of simple "wh" questions: "who," "what," "where," "when"
- develops awareness of many past experiences (e.g., is shown photo of past event and remembers)
- recognizes that stories have a sequence or order
- has increased attention span of at least ten minutes for story reading
- recognizes names of familiar settings such as playground, store, etc.
- recognizes at least two to three colors when named
- knows age and holds up appropriate number of fingers when asked
- initiates "pretend" behaviors or play in communication

Thirty-six to forty months

- has more complex understanding of number concepts (e.g., "none of them," "all of them")

- knows the concept of the number "two"

- has increased knowledge of words that depict texture ("smooth," "rough," etc.)

- knows at least three to four colors

- knows several words that describe feelings ("sad," "grumpy," "happy," etc.)

- responds to personal questions appropriately, such as "What's your name?"

Forty to forty-four months (about three and one-half years)

- responds to verbal directions involving a variety of prepositions ("Put the ball in the box, Stand in front of the chair," etc.)

- understands comparatives such as "Which is bigger, a house or a car?"

- follows a variety of instructions even when the objects requested are not present

- understands more time concepts (day, night, etc.)

- follows a three- to four-part instruction spoken within a sentence

- knows "three" and "four" number concepts

- develops understanding of basic problem solving by responding appropriately to "If . . .what" questions (e.g., "If you crossed the street without looking, what might happen?")

Forty-four to forty-eight months (four years)

- recognizes approximately 2,500 words

- knows shapes when named (crosses, triangles, squares)

- uses deduction to guess name of hidden object when given language clues

- responds correctly to questions that depict categories (e.g., "What barks?")

- reacts pleasurably to stories filled with action

- identifies at least six capital letters

- may associate a given letter with the beginning letter of a familiar name
- comprehends physical needs (e.g., "What do you do when you feel sleepy?")

Forty-eight to fifty-four months (four and one-half years)

- has receptive vocabulary of up to 5,000 words
- understands the function of body parts (e.g., we see with our eyes and hear with our ears)
- expands understanding of a variety texture words ("smooth," "rough," "bumpy," etc.)
- identifies coins (penny, nickel, dime) when asked
- understands what common items are made of when asked (e.g., a window is made of glass)

Fifty-four to sixty months (five years)

- has receptive vocabulary of up to 7,000 words
- identifies number concepts of one through five
- begins to distinguish right versus left
- identifies all the basic colors

Language Development Guide B: The Growth of Expressive Language in Children from Birth to Five Years

This guide outlines the major developments in vocabulary, grammar, sentence length, and use of basic concepts that occur in childrens' *expressive* (spoken) language during the first five years of life.

Birth to two months

- frequent crying predominates, with vocalizations changing in strength and intensity (loud vs. soft)
- initiates random vocalizing other than crying, such as hiccups, throaty sounds, etc.

- makes vowel-like sounds ("e/eh" and "a/ah" are most frequent)
- cry becomes more specialized to indicate hunger, displeasure, etc.
- makes more pleasurable vocalizations such as cooing, gurgling, etc.
- infrequently coos the same syllable or sound repeatedly

Two to four months

- repeats the same sounds frequently (e.g., cooing, gooing)
- begins to combine two or more different syllables (such as "ah-goo")
- initiates some throaty sounds such as "k," "g," "ng"
- responds vocally to social surroundings involving himself or herself, such as being held, spoken to, etc.
- smiles when spoken to or when views primary caregiver
- laughs aloud to indicate pleasure
- continues to create vocalizations unrelated to crying; vocalizations vary in intensity and pitch
- babbles (consistently repeats a series of the same sound or syllable, particularly when alone, such as "ba, ba, ba")
- begins to use the bilabial sounds (sounds produced by the lips) such as "p," "b," "m"

Four to six months

- indicates by sound or gesture if he or she wants something to occur again
- ceases babbling in response to an interruption or vocal stimulation
- babbles directly to person, and initiates vocalizations to others
- vocalizes emotions to indicate pleasure or anger by making sounds other than crying
- makes gurgling or playful sounds when left alone or while playing
- responds to image in mirror by vocalizing
- begins to combine four or more different syllables at a time when vocalizing
- initiates additional vowel-like sounds to include "o" and "u"

Six to eight months

- responds to his or her name with a vocalization at least 50 percent of the time
- babbles with varying inflections
- babbles using two syllables (repetitions of two or more different sounds)
- babbles or vocalizes in sentencelike utterances, but with no use of true words
- infrequently reacts to music or song by "singing along" with no true words
- begins to use more sounds in babbling ("t" and "d" as well as "n," "w," "f," "v," and "l")
- gestural imitation: mimics gestural language games like pat-a-cake, peek-a-boo
- expressions take on a wordlike quality when child begins to label things with his or her own "language"

Eight to ten months

- number of consonants in babbling expands to include groups of sounds both short and long (e.g., "tata," "bibibibi," "upup")
- makes some appropriate use of gestural language (e.g., shakes head for "no")
- seeks attention through gestures, speech with no crying sounds
- sound imitation: in response to vocal stimulation by others, mimics or models different sounds
- mimics adult facial gestures such as tongue clicking, kissing movements of the lips, etc.
- infrequently uses exclamations like "uh-oh"
- speaks first word, usually the name of a person or toy closely related to the child's experiences (e.g., "ba" for ball or "dada" for daddy)
- uses brief sentencelike utterances (jargon speech) to convey meaning without true words

Ten to twelve months

- speaks at least two to three words independently, either clearly or unclearly
- repeats an activity after obtaining attention for it (parent smiles and claps after child vocalizes)
- begins to initiate speech gesture games like pat-a-cake independently
- reacts to songs and rhymes through vocalization
- uses sentencelike utterances and jargon to talk to toys and people and while playing alone
- word imitation: infrequently attempts to mimic new words

Twelve to fourteen months

- uses sentencelike utterances and jargon with some true words
- is able to use five or more words
- uses generalization whereby one word has several meanings
- makes needs known by combining vocalizations with pointing and gesturing
- says "bye-bye" with no outside prompting
- more consistently models and mimics words spoken to him or her

Fourteen to sixteen months

- more consistently produces speech sounds such as "t," "d," "n," "w," "f," "h"
- has a vocabulary of at least seven true words
- uses true words along with gestures to indicate needs
- intermixes jargon with emerging vocabulary of true words

Sixteen to eighteen months

- expressive vocabulary gradually expands to at least eight to ten words
- words gradually replace gestures as the primary mode of communication
- repeats words that were heard in others' conversations

- begins to use intonation changes with jargon (e.g., pitch change at the end of a sentence to indicate a question)
- continues to mix jargon with expressive vocabulary

Eighteen to twenty months

- has expressive vocabulary of at least ten to twenty words, primarily familiar objects and persons in the environment
- puts two words together to create combinations such as:

   noun + noun ("Mommy sock")

   verb + object ("Give ball")

   subject + verb ("Daddy go")

   noun phrase ("Pretty baby")

   prepositional phrase ("on chair")
- mimics environmental sounds such as "meow" for a cat
- continues to combine jargon with true words
- begins to label at least two to three familiar objects seen in pictures
- models or mimics some two- and three-word sentences
- gestures or speaks to indicate when pants are soiled or wet

Twenty to twenty-two months

- vocabulary expands to at least twenty to fifty words
- relates personal experiences using a combination of jargon and words
- creates simple utterances by creating two-word sentences (e.g., "go bye-bye")
- responds with "no" to many requests

Twenty-two to twenty-four months

- has expressive vocabulary of at least fifty to one hundred words
- continues to use two-word utterances, but grammar is undeveloped
- infrequently speaks in three-word sentences with incorrect grammar (e.g., "me go bye-bye")

- uses own name when referring to self
- labels at least five to ten pictures of objects
- jargon begins to be discarded and is replaced with more true words and sentences
- responds to questions by repeating a word to indicate affirmation or "yes" (such as "want to go play?" and child responds with "play")
- uses the word "more" consistently when making requests
- includes negation in utterances ("no bye-bye")
- uses words to indicate location such as "here," "there," "inside," etc.
- uses some pronouns, as well as verbs (action words), adjectives (descriptors), and nouns (persons, places, or things) in utterances

Twenty-four to twenty-eight months

- combines words to create two- and three-word sentences
- jargon speech replaced completely with true sentences
- vocabulary expands to between 200 and 300 words
- uses a pronoun ("I," "me," "myself") to refer to self rather than given name
- uses commands such as "get ball"
- labels the names of at least ten to fifteen pictures
- requests help for personal needs such as brushing teeth, toileting, etc.
- says the name of at least one color correctly

Twenty-eight to thirty-two months

- vocabulary expands to at least 500 to 600 words
- uses two-word noun and verb combinations (e.g., "dog bark")
- uses speech to declare intentions (what he or she anticipates doing)
- begins to speak of past experiences or events
- responds with first and last name when asked for name
- describes what he or she is doing while playing or engaged in activity

- responds appropriately to "what" or "where" questions such as "Where is your ball?"
- mimics nursery rhymes, finger plays, or simple songs
- repeats two or three numbers in order in imitation of speaker
- uses articles such as "a" and "the" appropriately
- uses irregular past tense verbs incorrectly, such as "I runned" for "I ran"
- understands what gender he or she is by responding appropriately when asked "Are you a boy or a girl?"

Thirty-two to thirty-six months (three years)

- vocabulary expands to at least 600 to 1,000 words
- speech is intelligible to the familiar listener at least half the time
- spontaneous sentence length expands to three to four words (generally subject + verb + object combinations, such as "Mommy read book," or noun phrases, such as "Mommy red dress"; child will imitate up to seven-word sentences
- labels at least thirty to forty pictures of common objects
- when shown pictures, uses an appropriate verb (action word) to describe the activity
- regularly relates past experiences or events
- words that depict quantity emerge ("three," "many," etc.)
- words that indicate time begin to emerge (e.g., "today," "tomorrow," "yesterday")
- labels one color correctly
- often uses regular plurals such as "cats"; irregular form is inconsistent (such as "mouses" for "mice")
- negation emerging: primarily "no" and "not"
- verb forms emerging:
    present progressive—"jumping"
    present tense—"jump"
    inconsistent third person singular—"jumps"
    inconsistent simple past tense—"jumped"

- "wh" questions emerging but are inconsistent
- conjunction "and" used consistently by age three
- prepositions emerge—usually "in," "on," "under" are first
- auxiliary verbs emerging, such as "am," "are," "is," "was," "were"
- adverbs emerging—primarily in the form of location ("put there") and space ("stand up")

Thirty-six to forty months

- says at least two words that describe actions (e.g., "fast," "slow")
- prepositions increase to at least three to four, first used as verb particles (e.g., "lie down," "stand up"), followed by prepositions of location such as "by," "between," "beside" and then "in front of," "in back of," "behind"
- uses words to describe what certain objects are used for
- begins to use words that depict opposites ("tall and short," "big and small," etc.)
- labels at least two to three colors
- counts in correct order up to three or four
- uses complex sentences with conjunctions such as "and," "but," etc.
- uses "wh" questions ("what," "where," "when"); "why" emerges later

Forty to forty-four months (about three and one-half years)

- uses pronouns to replace objects in sentences (e.g., "He hit them.")
- words used to depict quantity are more complex ("a little more," etc.)
- simple sentences are grammatically correct most of the time
- uses verbs to denote future tense (e.g., "I *will go* to school")
- questions include "how" or "why"
- uses possessive pronouns such as "his," "her," "hers," "their," "theirs," "our," "ours," "mine," "my," "your," "yours," "its"
- uses words to label categories of items (e.g., toys, food, animals)

- expands grammatical skills to include contractions (e.g., "there's" for "there is")
- labels up to four colors
- independently recites at least one rhyme, song, or jingle that relies on word repetition
- uses pictures to tell stories
- engages in self-talk, generally pretend or make-believe

Forty-four to forty-eight months (four years)

- spontaneous sentence length expanded to four to five words
- labels most colors
- uses sentences that demonstrate projection or imagination such as "I wonder what _____"
- uses a vocabulary of at least 1,500 words
- uses words to express feelings, such as "I feel happy"
- verbally counts from one to ten
- is intelligible at least 90 percent of the time to the familiar listener
- explains the function of items when asked "What are scissors for?" etc.
- responds to questions relating to time such as today, yesterday, tomorrow
- recognizes when information is incorrect and protests verbally
- by age four, uses most simple verb forms consistently (e.g., "jumps," "jumped," "jumping")
- by age four, conjunctions in used complex sentences include "because," "if," and "so"

Forty-eight to fifty-four months (four and one-half years)

- has expressive vocabulary of up to 2,000 words
- uses spontaneous sentences containing approximately five to six words per utterance
- counts from one to twenty in sequence
- uses socially common expressions (e.g., "I don't care")

- sentences are grammatically complete and verbally cor
  majority of the time
- asks a variety of questions
- uses language to control people or situations (e.g., "tie my shoe")
- uses pictures to "read" a story
- combines pretend with reality to create long stories expressed verbally
- use of irregular plurals emerges: "feet" vs. "feets" or "foots"

Fifty-four to sixty months (five years)
- has expressive vocabulary of at least 2,200 words
- average spontaneous sentence length of six to seven words
- uses verbal descriptions to identify pictures not labeled
- repeats verbatim and remembers a series of numbers out of sequence (auditory memory)
- is able to print simple words
- counts from one to thirty in order
- tells home address when asked
- seeks answers to meaningful and thought-provoking questions (e.g., "why did that happen?")
- consistently uses verbally complex and grammatically complete sentences

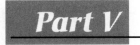

Part V

Issues of
the Voice

Voice defined: The involvement of the phonatory system (larynx and associated structures), respiratory system (breathing apparatus), and resonatory system (vibrating chambers or cavities) to produce audible sound.

41

How is a voice problem distinguished from a speech or language problem?

So far we have seen that speech, or articulation, is the motor act involving different organs and anatomical structures to clearly produce different sounds. Language is the symbolic system of words and word patterns we use to communicate with others. Voice, as distinct from speech and language, refers to how the vocal cords (sometimes commonly called the "voicebox"), the respiratory system (lungs, diaphragm, etc.), and the resonatory system (oral and nasal cavities, palate, etc.) work together to phonate, or create audible sound. Thus, when we communicate with spoken words, we combine the systems of the voice, speech or articulation, and language to express our thoughts.

Very simply, in order for phonation to occur, respiration (the breathing apparatus) will be the driving force (see Appendix A). Before we begin speaking, we inhale air. Upon exhalation, the airstream flows back through the top of the airway and sets the two vocal cords into vibration. This vocal cord vibration is what we hear as sound generated from the laryngeal area. If you hold your hand lightly over your throat, you can feel the vocal cords vibrating whenever you say a voiced sound such as "b," "d," "g," "v," or "z," and all vowels. Some of the sounds of our language do not involve the vibration or the vocal cords, such as "p," "t," "k," and "f" to name a few.

A child with a voicing problem will articulate sounds correctly and will show normal language development, but he may whisper rather than speak out clearly, or his speaking voice may sound unnatural or forced, or he may use his voice at pitch and loudness levels that are inappropriate or extreme for his age or sex or for the environment in which the voice is used.

Parent Strategy

All children experiment with their voices and may go through periods of speaking very softly, whispering, yelling, or using an unusual tone of voice. However, if these behaviors persist or become more pronounced, review the guidelines presented in question 44. If you remain concerned about your child's voice or voicing, consult a speech-language pathologist (SLP).

42

Explain why the vocal cords are important in producing voice.

The vocal cords serve many functions, but their relationship to pitch will be emphasized here. The vocal cords and their subsequent vibration are what produce the sound we know as voice. The rate or speed of vocal cord vibration is a product of the mass, length, and tension of the vocal cords, and it has the greatest impact on the pitch of the voice (how high or low the voice is). The loudness or intensity of the voice is a function of the amount of air pressure exerted from the lungs as well as the subsequent subglottal pressure that builds beneath the vocal cords.

As the mass or thickness of the vocal cords increases, vocal cord vibration is reduced, resulting in a lowered pitch. Decreased vocal cord mass results in an increased rate of vocal cord vibration, and thus a higher pitch. This explains why most women's voices are higher in pitch than most men's: most men have thicker vocal cords. Higher pitches are also related to increased vocal cord length (the thickness of the cords will decrease when the cords lengthen), and to increased tension in the vocal cords.

The vocal cords must be treated with reverence and care. They are quite sensitive to excessive tension, as well as unnatural and frequent extremes of pitch and loudness changes. As a result, development or growth of any organic pathology (e.g., nodules or polyps) is always a possibility (see question 49 and Appendix C).

Parent Strategy

Teach your child good vocal habits to properly care for the voice. Follow the recommendations given under the section for vocal hygiene and care in question 45.

43

What are the primary causes of a voice disorder?

Basically, the causes of voice problems in children can be categorized as either organic or functional. An organic cause has a neurological or medical basis, such as growths on the vocal cords that ultimately affect vibration. Organic sources generally have a slow onset, developing over periods ranging from several weeks to months or even years. However, some functional causes develop over a period of several weeks or months, similar to organic conditions.

Functional causes include any condition that cannot be explained by neurological or medical evidence. A functional voice problem is generally related to emotions or stress, and the onset is usually abrupt.

For example, adult patients have been known to become suddenly voiceless upon experiencing a psychologically traumatic incident.

At times it is difficult to make a clear distinction between an organic voice problem and a functional voice problem. For example, the modeling of poor voice standards in the environment (e.g., excessive yelling and screaming) can turn a functional voice disorder into an organic one if nodules develop on the vocal cords because of the excessive vocal abuse. Also, the presence of an organic condition (such as physical trauma or damage to the vocal mechanism) can create such psychic stress for the individual that the actual resulting voice disorder is far more severe than what the original organic condition would have caused. Finally, there may be ongoing contributing factors such as upper respiratory diseases and allergies, which will exacerbate an existing organic or functional voice disorder.

Parent Strategy

Whether the cause of the voice problem is functional or organic, its symptoms will affect the quality, intensity, pitch, or resonance of the voice. These are discussed in greater detail in question 44. If a voice evaluation is recommended, a speech-language pathologist and an ENT will determine whether the problem is functional or organic in nature and will provide treatment and suggestions for alleviating the cause as well as the symptoms of the difficulty.

44

What types of voice problems are commonly observed?

As mentioned above, four separate areas can be affected when the child has a voice disorder. These are the quality, intensity or loudness, pitch, and resonance of the voice.

Quality refers to any disturbance in the tone or voice at the vocal cord level. Observable difficulties to vocal quality include harshness, breathiness, and hoarseness. A harsh voice sounds quite rough and strained, and there is usually tension in the laryngeal area (throat). A harsh voice is often due to the forced production of phonation through tightly closed vocal cords. A breathy voice is whisperlike because of air escaping between the vocal cords, which are improperly closed while phonating (producing sound). A hoarse voice sounds husky and coarse, often accompanies the common cold, and has elements of both the harsh and breathy qualities.

Intensity refers to the loudness of the voice. When a voice is either too loud or too soft, this is considered to be an intensity difficulty. Often children who speak too loudly can be heard over the din of noise in the background and do not soften their voices even in quieter environments. A child with an excessively soft voice is constantly being told to speak up and probably tires of having to repeat herself.

Pitch is how low or high the voice sounds, and is a function both of the age and the sex of the child. For example, you would not expect a higher-pitched voice in a postpubescent male just as surely as you would not anticipate an excessively low pitch in a prepubescent female. Both boys and girls go through a period of voice change that is well under way by age fourteen or fifteen, in which the pitch level drops for both sexes.

Resonance refers to the vibrating chambers and anatomical structures that change how the voice will sound once produced. The most common resonators for the voice are the oral cavity (inside mouth) and the nasal cavity (inside nose). Two of the most common resonance problems are related to nasality. These include hyponasality (not enough involvement of the nasal cavity during voice productions), which sounds similar to someone with a head cold, and hypernasality (too much involvement of the nasal cavity during voice production). Someone who is hypernasal may sound as if she is "talking through her nose."

Parent Strategy

The following are suggestions when encountering any of the above in your child:

Quality: Hoarseness is one of the most commonly observed vocal problems in children. When hoarseness is observed in the presence of a cold, there is generally no need for concern. However, if the hoarseness persists beyond ten days to two weeks, professional evaluation may be necessary. Some children develop hoarseness as a result of misuse (screaming or yelling) or overuse (talking for excessive amounts of time). Chronic hoarseness, harshness, or breathiness can be a source of concern. For hoarseness, consult a speech-language pathologist and an ear, nose, and throat specialist (ENT) for an evaluation. Also, ensure good vocal hygiene by following the recommendations given in question 45.

Intensity: Children who often speak excessively loudly or softly should be evaluated by an audiologist for investigation of any hearing loss. The hearing mechanism is our source of self-monitoring. When we speak to someone else, we listen to monitor the accuracy of what we are saying. We can then change what is said if we feel the information needs to be altered. In the case of intensity or loudness levels, if a hearing loss is present, the child will have difficulty adequately monitoring the intensity of her own voice. If no hearing loss is present, you may wish to consult a speech-language pathologist for an opinion, and follow the recommendations given in the vocal hygiene program.

Pitch: All of us have a habitual pitch level—the level at which we normally speak. However, this level may not be optimal for our individual anatomical vocal structure. Optimal pitch is the level at which the voice is produced with the least amount of effort, with an absence of any tension. When someone's habitual pitch level approximates what is optimal, there is less likelihood that a voice disorder will develop. However, if someone routinely attempts to speak at a higher or lower pitch level than is optimal, a voice disorder can result. Note that it is excessive speaking at these unnatural levels that will create difficulties, not random changes in pitch levels. If you are concerned about your child's pitch, particularly if it appears inappropriate for his or her age and gender, consult a speech-language pathologist.

Resonance: Sometimes a child can develop hypernasality as a result of an adenoidectomy (removal of the tonsils, or adenoids). Hypernasality can also be the result of other medical or anatomical conditions, such as clefts of the hard or soft palates, and can also be a learned vocal style. Hyponasality often results from a nasal obstruction such as a deviated septum, enlarged adenoids, or nasal polyps. All these conditions can cause a lack of nasal resonance when the nasal consonants "m," "n," and "ng" are produced, and the child may sound as if she has a head cold. If you suspect a resonance difficulty, consult a speech-language pathologist.

45

What can I do to teach my child to take care of his voice?

Children have to be taught to take care of everything that belongs to them. Their voices are no different; they require proper care. In order to use their voices properly, children must have proper models and be taught what is good versus improper use of their voices.

Parent Strategy

To encourage your child to use his voice properly, teach him to follow these guidelines for good vocal hygiene (portions adapted from Wilson 1987, 165):

1. Speak easily and smoothly, with the muscles involved in speaking (those of the face, throat, neck, shoulders) kept as relaxed as possible

2. When speaking with others, keep within a reasonable distance of the listener: two to three feet. This makes it unnecessary to shout across the room.

3. When in a group of people, stay within the center of the group. This will enable you to be heard without having to talk loudly. Also, get the listener's attention before beginning to speak.

4. When you have an upper respiratory infection, such as a cold or laryngitis, avoid talking too much.

5. During cold weather, avoid breathing through your mouth.

6. Some medications, such as antihistamines, can dry out the mucous membranes in the mouth and throat. This can create the need to clear the throat frequently. Routinely drink water to lessen the effects of these types of medications. Also, use of a humidifier in the house is helpful in remediating the dryness.

7. Do not attempt to compete with loud machinery or other loud noises when speaking.

8. Wear seat belts in autos. In the event of an accident or sudden stop, you could hit the dashboard, resulting in trauma to the larynx and vocal mechanism.

9. Speak at a pitch level that is optimal or most natural for you. If you walk around imitating Minnie Mouse day after day, chances are you will develop a vocal problem. The same is true if you routinely use an abnormally low pitch.

10. Avoid airborne laryngeal irritants such as smoke and dust. Alcohol, caffeine, and tobacco products also irritate the vocal cords. Avoid ingestion of milk products and chocolate if recovering from an upper respiratory condition, sore throat, or laryngitis, because these products tend to create a need to clear the throat. Drink plenty of water.

46

What are some common vocal abuses or misuses that my child should avoid?

Vocal abuse is the result of poor vocal hygiene, and it can include any activity that has a traumatic effect on the vocal cords. It is natural that many children are going to scream and yell while playing. However, it is when these behaviors turn into a habitual pattern that the behavior can be considered abusive to the voice. Some of the common vocal abuses include:

1. Excessive coughing or throat clearing. When an individual either coughs or clears the throat, the vocal cords slam together, with the vocal cords vibrating explosively. If this is done excessively, eventually sores or other physical changes will develop on the vocal cords as a result. Monitor the use of antihistamines for allergy control, because these can create excessive dryness in the lining for the mouth and throat and thus create a need for throat clearing.

2. Speaking while lifting or exerting pressure. When an individual attempts to lift a heavy object, the vocal cords automatically come together to close the airway tightly. If speaking is attempted while

one is lifting heavy items, phonation will be strained and will place undue stress on the vocal cords. Children also use strained vocalizations in an attempt to imitate the sounds of airplanes, guns, lasers, or cars. If these vocalizations are excessive, vocal cord irritation is a likely result.

3. Improper uses of the voice, including shouting, screaming, excessively loud laughter, reverse phonation (speaking on inhalation instead of exhalation), cheering, and excessive talking. Singing can be a traumatic event to the vocal cords if performed at an inappropriate pitch or loudness level, or if the person is suffering from an upper respiratory condition.

4. Use of a forced whisper to talk. Just as an excessively loud voice can create a voice disorder, so can use of whispering when done habitually. When someone whispers, the vocal cords come together to make contact so that phonation or vocal cord vibration can occur (just as when we prepare to speak at a normal intensity level). However, when the person whispers, the vocal cords are just slightly parted so that enough airstream flows through the vocal cords. This escaping air is what causes the hiss that accompanies the whisper. But to maintain the vocal cords in this position requires a great deal of stress on the cords, since it is a rather unnatural state for speaking.

5. Abusing the vocal cords when they are weakened by illness or infection. The vocal cords are extremely vulnerable to damage if used over a long period of time, particularly if they are reddened and swollen from allergies or an upper respiratory infection. Thus, if damage can occur to the cords during normal speaking conditions in this situation, it is highly likely that damage will ensue if the cords are abused by screaming, yelling, singing, and so on.

Vocal misuse is the incorrect use of pitch or loudness in voice production. Vocal misuse that is not corrected can result in vocal abuse. Some examples of vocal misuse include:

1. Speaking at an unnatural pitch level (either too high or too low). This again causes the vocal cords to constantly perform in an unnatural way, and thus creates strain and stress on the vocal cords.

2. Speaking too loudly on a frequent basis. This usually occurs while in noisy environments such as around heavy machinery, motorcycles, excessively loud music, or any environment that has a high background noise level. Any time there is an increase in vocal loudness, there is an increase in the amount of laryngeal tension, and thus a greater chance of traumatizing the vocal cords.

Parent Strategy

Follow the guidelines for the vocal hygiene program outlined in question 45.

47

What is laryngitis, and what causes it?

The most common form of laryngitis is called chronic nonspecific laryngitis. Hoarseness, a lowered pitch level, and vocal fatigue are the most common complaints of sufferers with this condition. The most frequent causes of chronic laryngitis are cigarette smoking, vocal abuse or misuse, industrial airborne toxins or pollutants, or drainage of a chronic sinus problem. In some instances, persistent mouth breathing (which dries out and irritates the lining of the mouth and throat) and abuse of mouthwashes and gargles can lead to laryngitis (Prater and Swift 1984, 79).

Parent Strategy

Management of laryngitis will depend on the suspected cause of laryngeal irritation. If the difficulty is inhalation of cigarette smoke, the parent may be asked to limit smoking to one room in the house or outdoors to prevent laryngeal irritation in the children. If sinusitis is the suspected cause, usually medical management is necessary to control the sinusitis and thus drainage over the vocal cords. If vocal misuse or abuse is the concern, a vocal hygiene program is in order. Finally, limit intake of products that contain caffeine, chocolate, and milk; and have your child drink water routinely. A period of vocal rest is also in order, in which the child's amount of daily talking is reduced until the laryngitis has subsided. See question 50.

48

Why are screaming and yelling so damaging to the voice?

As mentioned previously, any vocal behavior when performed in excess can create a potential voice problem. If the vocal cords are stressed enough either through improper use of vocal intensity (screaming, shouting, whispering, etc.), vocal pitch levels (higher or lower than anatomically optimal for the individual), or development of certain habits (excessive coughing or throat clearing), the vocal cords will eventually evidence the strain. As with any structure that is overused, the vocal cords will tire and gradually show the wear of abuse. Physical changes will then begin to develop on the cords, usually in the form of vocal nodules (small bumps on the cords), vocal polyps, or contact ulcers (sores).

Parent Strategy

Follow the suggestions given for the vocal hygiene program if your child appears to be engaging in excessive yelling, screaming, or loud talking.

49

My child has been diagnosed with vocal nodules. What are these, and how will they affect his voice?

Vocal nodules are small growths that develop on the vocal cords, often because of vocal abuse or misuse, and are one of the most common voice disorders in children (see Appendix C). The incidence of vocal nodules is more frequent in boys than in girls. However, in adulthood the condition is more prevalent in women than in men (Prater and Swift 1984, 83).

When vocal nodules are present, the voice will sound hoarse and breathy, with a lowered pitch level. Other symptoms may include an improved vocal quality in the morning hours, with a gradual worsening of the vocal condition as the day progresses.

Parent Strategy

If the vocal nodules are immature and nonfibrous, voice therapy will generally aid in reducing or eliminating them. However, fibrous mature nodules will generally not respond to voice therapy techniques. Surgical removal is in order in these instances. An evaluation by an ear, nose, and throat specialist (ENT) will aid in determining the type of vocal nodules, and thus the corresponding management.

It is essential to remember that good vocal hygiene is the key to preventing the development and recurrence of vocal nodules. Thus, if an individual were to have vocal nodules removed, the removal would be in vain if the child did not receive voice therapy to change the vocal habits that created the nodules in the first place. To manage vocal nodules successfully, the following steps are suggested:

1. An evaluation by an ENT *and* a speech-language pathologist.

2. A period of vocal rest or a reduction in the amount of time the voice is used during the day.

3. A program of vocal hygiene supervised by a speech-language pathologist (see question 45).

4. Voice therapy by a certified speech-language pathologist to eliminate the abusive vocal behaviors. If a program of voice therapy is not instituted to eliminate the abusive behaviors, the nodules will simply return after being removed because the source of the problem was never addressed.

50

When would a period of vocal rest be warranted?

Vocal rest implies that the use of the vocal mechanism would be modified on a part- or full-time basis for a specific period of time. Vocal rest is generally indicated for a period of four to seven days, up to a maximum of two weeks. A program of vocal rest is usually advised under the following conditions (Prater and Swift 1984, 101):

1. Any type of surgery involving the larynx (vocal mechanism) or vocal cords. Mandatory vocal rest is generally indicated in these situations to prevent irritation to the vocal structures during the healing process.

2. Abuse-related conditions. Chronic laryngitis and vocal nodules are often the result of vocal abuse: excessive shouting, speaking at an unnatural pitch level, excessive coughing, and so on. Thus, vocal rest and therefore cessation of abusive activity would aid the structures of the vocal mechanism.

Parent Strategy

Requiring a child to undergo a period of vocal rest is difficult at best but certainly attainable. Children who are candidates for vocal rest are selected carefully under the supervision of a speech-language pathologist. If after seven days the program appears to be having no success, it should be discontinued.

It is essential to keep in mind that parental and familial support is necessary for the success of any vocal rest program, or any behavioral change. Also, it may be necessary to develop a reward system that will aid in motivating the child to stay on the program. For example, once per week the family could go swimming, go to a movie, and so on. If the reward involves the child's siblings and parents, the vocal rest program will be more likely to succeed.

In the suggestions outlined below, the vocal rest program is for a modified rather than a complete vocal rest. The goal is to modify or reduce the amount of talking over a seven-day period by at least one-half or more. Although some talking is allowed under the modified approach, it can occur only under the following six conditions (Prater and Swift 1984, 105–106):

1. Quiet talking is permitted to family members in the morning before school. No forced speech or whispering.

2. Talking to large groups of people (e.g., giving speeches, acting in plays) encourages increased vocal loudness and is not allowed. Singing is permitted. However, the child is expected to answer questions in class.

3. Absolutely no talking is permitted during recess, lunch, or PE class. These environments often have a high level of background noise and require the child to speak at louder levels to be heard. If no speaking at all is allowed in these conditions, the child is not placed in the predicament of ever having to raise her intensity or loudness level.

4. Talking quietly is permitted after school to family members, but only for a short period of time. After this, no more talking is allowed until dinnertime.

5. During mealtimes, the child is allowed to talk quietly to the entire family. All family members should be encouraged to model quiet talking habits to set the tone of the evening meal. If the family's conversational style at mealtime is one of verbal competition, children may try to engage the attention of parents by talking more loudly than anyone else. This should be strongly discouraged because it will support the child's abusive vocal patterns. Positive parental and family role models for speaking are essential.

6. Limit the amount of the child's talking for the remainder of the evening as much as possible.

For a child who needs vocal rest, a whistle is very useful for getting the attention of siblings, parents, or playmates when in a noisy environment. This eliminates the need for the child to shout above the din to be heard. The whistle can be worn around the neck at all times during the period of vocal rest; however, the child has to be taught to use it with discretion, and generally in situations where the noise level necessitates its usage.

Although a whistle can certainly be helpful in a noisy environment, I strongly suggest to the parent that there is no substitute for developing good vocal behaviors. Teach your child that if she needs to get the attention of a teacher or a playmate in a group or noisy environment, it is essential to pay attention to the distance between the speaker and listener. The closer this distance is, the less likely the child will be required to yell to get attention, particularly in noisy situations. If the child is within two to three feet of her listener, she can usually also manage to be within the listener's visual field and can also gain his or her attention by touching an arm or hand. Once it is clear that she has the listener's attention, she can begin speaking.

Finally, remember to engage the assistance of a speech-language pathologist before attempting any vocal rest program.

Closing Remarks

If, after reviewing the fifty questions answered in this book, you believe your child may have a speech or language problem that is not developmental in nature, contact a speech-language pathologist as soon as possible. If you need assistance in determining whether your child needs speech-language therapy, contact the American Speech-Language and Hearing Association (ASHA) or your local state organization. (See Part VI for a list of resources for parents.)

Begin by reviewing the section on legislation in the back of this book. Public schools are required by law to provide "support services," including speech-language therapy, for eligible students from ages three through twenty-one. Eligibility is defined by state laws that determine whether a student is considered communication-disordered, or by other defined parameters. To find out whether your child is eligible, contact your state speech and hearing association (see Part VI for a listing in your area), your state education department, or the U.S. Department of Education. Your local public library may have copies of the federal laws listed in this book. If not, they can be obtained via interlibrary loan from another library in the state, particularly a university-sponsored law library. Check the Internet as well.

Eligibility for speech-language therapy in the public schools varies from state to state, depending on how each state interprets the federal guidelines and chooses its terminology. Find out from your local speech and hearing organization or your state's Department of Education what the specific elegibility requirements are, not only for your state, but for your local school district. I have found different criteria in school districts within a single state.

If you suspect that your child has a speech or language difficulty that is not developmental, you may request a speech-language screening from your school. The referral does not have to come from your child's classroom teacher or from anyone else at the school. If the screening indicates a problem, the school speech-language pathologist (SLP) will complete a full evaluation, which takes up to two hours in most cases. The evaluation will pinpoint areas of strength and of weakness, with recommendations for treatment. Treatment will generally be provided on-site by the school SLP. In rural schools, services are often provided by a board of cooperative services that travels from school to school.

Whether the school is urban or rural, once your child is deemed eligible for speech-language therapy, the school is required by law to provide treatment. If an SLP is not available in the school, it is the school's responsibility to contract with an outside source, generally a private practitioner. Know your rights as parents under the federal laws described in this book.

Whether you select a speech-language pathologist (SLP) through the school system or independently, make sure to choose one who is licensed or certified within your state. Requirements differ by state. SLPs are required to have a minimum of a master's degree, with a certificate of clinical competence issued by the national association (ASHA). In addition, keep the following in mind when selecting a speech-language pathologist:

1. Both you and your child should meet in person with the SLP before making any commitments toward therapy. Develop your own perceptions as to whether this individual will mesh on an interpersonal level with your child. A qualified therapist can come highly recommended by friends or family and have glowing academic credentials. But if your child does not connect with that

therapist, you may be spending valuable time and money on ineffective treatment. Child-therapist rapport is essential.

2. Select a therapist who is willing to provide a parent-child treatment program for home use. The therapist will be spending as little as thirty minutes to one hour per session with your child, so follow-up of those skills at home is essential to a successful treatment program. In addition, always request copies of the speech-language evaluation and the subsequent therapy goals and objectives. An effective therapist will develop a *written* home program from this evaluation for the parent and child outlining the goals of treatment, as well as practical activities for home use to accomplish those goals.

3. Don't be shy about speaking up. If you are unclear about why the therapist is working on a certain goal or the activities used to accomplish that goal, ask questions. Make a point to spend at least five minutes of your therapy time to confer with the therapist, and ask to observe therapy sessions periodically.

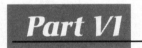

Part VI

Resources for Parents

Organizations and Associations

This list is not all-inclusive, but represents some of the organizations that I have drawn on over the years. I strongly suggest a trip to the library to use the Internet or one of the many databases (such as ERIC) now available.

Alexander Graham Bell Association for the Deaf (AGBA)
3417 Volta Place NW
Washington, DC 20007
(202) 337-5220 (Voice/TDD)

An association to assist hearing-impaired and deaf persons and their families. Excellent resources available for parents and children.

American Speech-Language and Hearing Association (ASHA)
10801 Rockville Pike
Rockville, MD 20852
(301) 897-5700 (Voice/TDD)
(800) 638-8255

The national association for speech-language pathologists and audiologists. ASHA will provide information regarding language, articulation, voice, stuttering, auditory processing, and hearing issues. ASHA will also have a current listing of the state speech-language and hearing associations for those interested in issues that pertain to a particular state.

Council for Exceptional Children (CEC)
1920 Association Drive
Reston, VA 20191-1589
(703) 620-3660

CEC is the largest international professional organization dedicated to improving educational outcomes for students with disabilities and the gifted.

Educational Resources Information Center (ERIC)
Clearinghouse on Elementary and Early Childhood Education
University of Illinois
805 West Pennsylvania Avenue
Urbana, IL 61801-4897
(800) 583-4135
(217) 333-1386

This is a national information system providing access to more than 850,000 abstracts of documents and articles on education. There are sixteen different clearinghouses for specific subjects. The Clearinghouse on Elementary and Early Childhood Education is just one of these.

John Tracy Clinic
806 West Adams Boulevard
Los Angeles, CA 90007
(800) 522-4582

Provides correspondence courses for parents of hearing-impaired or deaf children at no charge. Excellent materials and activities for the infant and preschooler (from birth to age five) in the areas of communication, general development, and so on. The program's mission is to offer emotional support, education, guidance, and encouragement.

Learning Disabilities Association of America (LDA)
4156 Library Road
Pittsburgh, PA 15234
Attention: Jean Peterson
(412) 341-1515

Founded in 1964 as a nonprofit organization to support parents and professionals who work with the learning disabled, this is an advocacy group that increases public awareness and disseminates information about learning disabilities.

National Information Center for Handicapped Children and Youth (NICHCY)
P.O. Box 1492
Washington, DC 20013
(800) 695-0285

Provides free information to interested parties helping children and youth with disabilities achieve their potential (speech and/or language disorders are considered disabilities). Services include responses to specific questions, referrals to other sources, general information packets, current publications, and technical assistance.

National Institute for the Deaf and Other Communication Disorders (NIDCD)
Information Clearinghouse
One Communication Avenue
Bethesda, MD 20892-3456
(800) 241-1044

A clearinghouse to provide information to consumers regarding deafness as well as communication disorders. Good resource for literature and information suitable for parents.

The Orton Dyslexia Society
Chester Building, Suite 382
8600 LaSalle Road
Baltimore, MD 21286-2044
(301) 296-0232
(800) 222-3123

Organization for persons with dyslexia and reading disabilities. Provides probrams, research, and publications on specific language disabilities.

SKI-HI Institute
Department of Communicative Disorders
Utah State University
Logan, UT 84322-1900
(801) 752-4601

A home intervention program for parents to work with their hearing-impaired or deaf child. Excellent activities for parents to work on language, communication, and auditory training; also information on understanding hearing impairments and deafness.

Stuttering Foundation of America
P.O. Box 11749
Memphis, TN 38111-0749
(800) 992-9392

An excellent organization for stutterers and parents of stutterers. Provides a tremendous number of resources and valuable publications important to adult stutterers and to parents of children who stutter.

The Voice Foundation
1721 Pine Street
Philadelphia, PA 19103
(215) 735-7999

A foundation dedicated to issues pertaining to the voice and voice disorders.

State Speech-Language-Hearing Associations

These associations will have information pertaining to issues in your state regarding speech-language and related services.

Speech and Hearing Association of Alabama
1248 Cottonwood Circle
Auburn, AL 36830
(205) 844-9600

Alaska Speech-Language-Hearing Association
P.O. Box 1803
Bethel, AK 99559
(907) 543-3690

Arizona Speech-Language-Hearing Association
1010 East McDowell Road, Suite 201
Phoenix, AZ 85006
(602) 254-6041

Arkansas Speech-Language-Hearing Association
P.O. Box 3835
Little Rock, AR 72203
(501) 450-5479

California Speech-Language-Hearing Association
825 University Avenue
Sacramento, CA 95825
(916) 921-1568, (310) 603-4835

Colorado Speech-Language-Hearing Association
1325 South Colorado Boulevard, Suite B401
Denver, CO 80222
(303) 753-1221, (303) 492-5375

Connecticut Speech-Language-Hearing Association
213 Back Lane
Newington, CT 06111
(203) 666-6900

Delaware Speech-Language-Hearing Association
P.O. Box 7383
Newark, DE 19714-7383
(302) 655-7784

District of Columbia Speech-Language-Hearing Association
P.O. Box 91016
Washington, DC 20090-1016
(202) 994-2177

Florida Language, Speech and Hearing Association
P.O. Box 10523
Tallahassee, FL 32302
(904) 222-1907, (813) 972-8449

Georgia Speech-Language-Hearing Association
P.O. Box 6708
Athens, GA 30604
(706) 613-0144, (404) 972-4938

Hawaii Speech-Language-Hearing Association
P.O. Box 1303
Kailua, HI 96734
(808) 396-8437, (808) 261-3234

Idaho Speech, Language and Hearing Association
2315 North 12th Street
Coeur D'Alene, ID 83814
(208) 765-5437

Illinois Speech-Language-Hearing Association
435 North Michigan Avenue
Suite 1717
Chicago, IL 60611
(312) 644-0828, (309) 794-7583

Indiana Speech-Language-Hearing Association
P.O. Box 984
Noblesville, IN 46060
(317) 773-3219, (219) 425-3728

Iowa Speech-Language-Hearing Association
520 35th Street
Des Moines, IA 50312
(515) 274-5918, (319) 338-1911

Kansas Speech-Language-Hearing Association
3900 17th Street
Great Bend, KS 67530
(316) 793-6550, (913) 764-1770

Kentucky Speech-Language-Hearing Association
366 Waller Avenue, Suite 113
Lexington, KY 40504
(606) 277-2446, (606) 281-0181

Louisiana Speech-Language-Hearing Association
8550 United Plaza Boulevard
Suite 1001
Baton Rouge, LA 70809
(504) 922-4600

Maine Speech-Language-Hearing Association
510 Main Street
Gorham, ME 04038
(207) 839-4007

Maryland Speech-Language-Hearing Association
P.O. Box 234
Columbia, MD 21045
(800) 622-6742

Massachusetts Speech-Language-Hearing Association
518 North Main Sreet
Randolph, MA 02368
(617) 986-8177

Michigan Speech-Language-Hearing Association
855 Grove Sreet
East Lansing, MI 48823
(517) 332-5691

Minnesota Speech-Language-Hearing Association
P.O. Box 26115
St. Louis Park, MN 55426
(612) 935-5057

Mississippi Speech-Language-Hearing Association
P.O. Box 5361
Fondren Station
Jackson, MS 39296
(601) 266-5232

Missouri Speech-Language-Hearing Association
200 East Market
Warrensburg, MO 64093
(816) 747-8666

Montana Speech-Language-Hearing Association
Box 372
Hamilton, MT 59840
(406) 363-2228

Nebraska Speech-Language-Hearing Association
1033 K Street
Lincoln, NB 68508
(402) 476-9573

Nevada Speech-Language-Hearing Association
77 Pringle Way
Reno, NV 89520
(702) 328-4963

New Hampshire Speech-Language-Hearing Association
Box 7202
Concord Heights Station
Concord, NH 03301
(603) 673-5250

New Jersey Speech-Language-Hearing Association
2 Greentree Center
Suite 225, Box 955
Marlton, NJ 08053
(609) 985-2878

New Mexico Speech-Language-Hearing Association
P.O. Box 53580
Albuquerque, NM 87153
(505) 281-8465

New York State Speech-Language-Hearing Association
48 Howard Sreet
Albany, NY 12207
(518) 463-5272

North Carolina Speech-Language-Hearing Association
P.O. Box 28359
Raleigh, NC 27611
(919) 833-3984

North Dakota Speech-Language-Hearing Association
P.O. Box 5175
Grand Forks, ND 58206
(701) 780-2439

Ohio Speech and Hearing Association
9331 South Union Road
Miamisburg, OH 45342
(513) 866-4972

Oklahoma Speech-Language-Hearing Association
P.O. Box 53217
Oklahoma City, OK 73152
(405) 769-7329

Oregon Speech-Language-Hearing Association
P.O. Box 523
1270 Chemeketa St NE
Salem, OR 97308
(503) 370-7019

Pennsylvania Speech-Language-Hearing Association
100 High Tower Boulevard
Suite 302
Pittsburgh, PA 15205
(215) 393-1703

Rhode Island Speech-Language-Hearing Association
P.O. Box 9241
Providence, RI 02940
(401) 724-0550

South Carolina Speech-Language-Hearing Association
3008 Millwood Avenue
Columbia, SC 29205
(803) 252-5646

South Dakota Speech-Language-Hearing Association
210 W. Main
Beresford, SD 57004
(605) 763-5012

Tennesee Association of Audiologists and Speech-Language Pathologists
530 Church Sreet
Suite 501
Nashville, TN 37219
(615) 254-3687

Texas Speech-Language-Hearing Association
P.O. Box 140046
Austin, TX 78714
(512) 452-4571

Utah Speech-Language-Hearing Association
10720 Dimple Dell Drive
Sandy, UT 84092
(801) 561-3400

Vermont Speech-Language-Hearing Association
Rural Route 1, Box 3094
Rutland, VT 05701
(802) 775-5196

Speech and Hearing Association of Virginia
P.O. Box 35653
Richmond, VA 23235
(804) 379-8441

Washington Speech and Hearing Association
2033 Sixth Avenue
Suite 804
Seattle, WA 98121
(206) 441-6020

West Virginia Speech-Language-Hearing Association
Route 1, Box 32
West Hamlin, WV 25571
(304) 824-3032

Wisconsin Speech-Language-Hearing Association
330 East Lakeside Street
P.O. Box 1109
Madison, WI 53701
(800) 545-0640

Wyoming Speech-Language-Hearing Association
1103 Mill Street
Laramie, WY 82070
(307) 766-3985

Overseas Association of Communication Sciences (OSACS)
Argonner Elementary School
Unit 20235
APO, AE 09165
Hanau, Germany
(431) 269-2697, ext. 379

Puerto Rico Organizacion Puertorriquena de Patologia del Hablo-Lenguaje y Audiologia
P.O. Box 20147
Rio Piedras, Puerto Rico 00928-0147

Books and Materials

Chinaberry Book Service
2780 Via Orange Way, Suite B
Spring Valley, CA 91978
(800) 776-2242

An excellent and comprehensive resource for parents. Catalogs include detailed descriptions of current children's books on the market, with book selection guide indicating the suitable developmental levels. Parent feedback is also included on different book selections based on personal experience. I strongly recommend at least getting the catalog to use as a guide when purchasing suitable books for children.

HELP Activity Guides
Author: Setsu Furuno
The VORT Corporation
P.O. Box 60132
Palo Alto, CA 94306
(415) 322-8282

I highly recommend these two books, one on child development from birth to age three and the second for ages three to six. These guides contain developmental charts and activities designed to assist development in cognition and receptive language, expressive language, fine and gross motor skills, self-help, and social-emotional skills. An excellent and comprehensive resource that is invaluable for all parents. Request a catalog for other products available through this company.

Hartley, Ruth E., and Robert M. Goldenson. 1963. *The Complete Book of Children's Play.* New York: Harper & Row.
Children's play from infancy on. Ideas on household items to use as play material.

Scheffler, Hannah Nuba. 1983. *Resources for Early Childhood: An Annotated Bibliography and Guide for Educators, Librarians, Health Care Professionals, and Parents.* **New York: Garland Publishing.**
A comprehensive listing of resources available in early childhood development, many of them helpful for parents.

Strichart, Stephen S., and Charles T. Mangrum II. 1993. *Teaching Study Strategies to Students with Learning Disabilities.* **Needham Heights, Mass.: Allyn and Bacon.**
These strategies are applicable and helpful for all students at the middle school and high school levels, not just the learning disabled. Strategies are included in the areas of time management, note taking, memory, and taking tests, to name a few. Very practical and easy to use. Could be adapted for the elementary age level.

Legislation

Contact your local librarian for the specifics on these laws. The Internet also has a multitude of information pertaining to special education and disabilities legislation.

1973

Section 504 of the Rehabilitation Act of 1973
Eliminates discrimination on the basis of handicap in any program or activity receiving Federal financial assistance.

1975

The Education for All Handicapped Children Act (P.L. 94-142)
Requires public schools to provide free appropriate public education for school-aged handicapped children and young adults (to age twenty-one), including special education and related services (e.g., speech therapy), regular education, and specially designed vocational education if needed.

1987

P.L. 457

Extends all the rights and protections of P.L. 94-142 to handicapped children ages three through five years, effective 1990–1991.

Appendix A

Cross-Section of the Head Showing the Principal Speech Organs

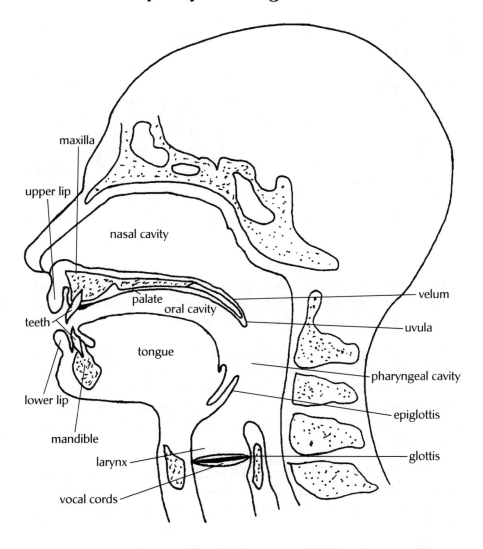

Appendix B

Cross-Section of the Ear

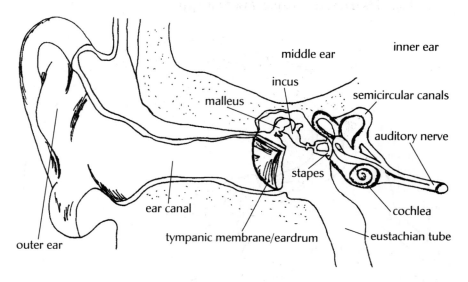

The outer ear includes the visible portion of the ear, the ear canal, and the eardrum, or tympanic membrane. Sound waves are conducted down the canal and set the eardrum into vibration.

The middle ear is an irregularly shaped chamber about the size of a garden pea. The rear surface of the eardrum is attached to three tiny bones, or ossicles (the malleus, incus, and stapes). The movements of the ossicular chain transmit the sound waves into mechanical energy. This energy is transmitted across the middle ear chamber to the oval window of the inner ear.

The inner ear is also known as the labyrinth because it contains many chambers and canals. The inner ear contains the semicircular canals (used for balance), the cochlea (which contains nerve endings for the auditory nerve to transmit signals to the brain), and the vestibule (which connects the cochlea to the semicircular canals).

Appendix C

Vocal Cords and Organic Pathology

(Viewed from above looking down into the airway, or trachea)

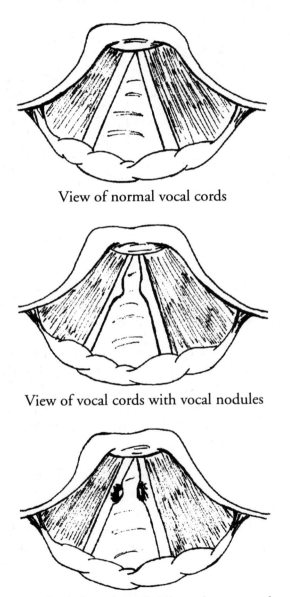

View of normal vocal cords

View of vocal cords with vocal nodules

View of vocal cords with bilateral contact ulcer

Glossary

(Terms in SMALL CAPS are defined elsewhere in this glossary.)

acoustic: Relating to the sensation or perception of sound.

affricate: A phoneme, or sound, created from combining a plosive with a fricative. Examples include "ch" and "j."

alveolar ridge: A ridge of bone located behind the teeth.

anterior crossbite: The relationship between the upper and lower teeth whereby the lower teeth are wider than, or on the outside of, the upper teeth when the two sets are in contact with each other.

articulation: The ability to speak clearly and intelligibly. Involves primarily the structures and actions of the tongue, lips, teeth, and throat.

attention deficit disorder (ADD): A complex host of behaviors dominated by the inability to stay focused or to attend to tasks.

audiogram: A diagram used to depict the results of a hearing test or screening. The audiogram outlines the levels at which the individual is able to hear when tested with certain loudness levels and frequencies.

audiologist: A professional trained to diagnose and treat hearing difficulties.

auditory: Pertaining to hearing.

auditory discrimination: The ability to use hearing to discriminate between similar-sounding words, phonemes, or phrases.

auditory memory: The ability to recall information that was heard.

auditory pathway: The neurological connections for hearing connecting the INNER EAR to the brain.

auditory processing: The ability to attach meaning to an acoustic message.

auditory processing deficit: Difficulty with the auditory processing system. See INFORMATION CAPACITY DEFICIT, INTERMITTENT AUDITORY PERCEPTION, NOISE BUILD-UP, RETENTION DEFICIT, SLOW RISE TIME.

block: A complete disruption in the flow of speech, generally accompanied by struggle within the muscles of the face and larynx during a stuttering moment.

breathiness: A vocal quality characterized by air escaping through the vocal cords.

cerebral cortex: The part of the brain whose main function is to process motor and sensory information.

cerebral palsy: A group of neurological disorders that result from insult or injury to the brain, generally at birth, and affect the motor skills and coordination.

cleft lip or palate: Failure of the two halves of the lip or palate to grow together during the embryological period (between the sixth and ninth week of gestation).

cognition: The conscious knowing of information through the use of higher-level functions, thoughts, and ideas.

conductive hearing loss: Hearing loss associated with reduced ability to receive sound through the middle ear (e.g., due to blockage). See also PERIPHERAL HEARING LOSS, SENSORINEURAL HEARING LOSS.

congenital: Present at birth.

decibel (dB): The unit of measure for loudness or intensity of sound.

developmental apraxia: An inability to sequence sounds to produce words, generally manifested as a severe articulation disorder.

developmental stuttering: A period of normal dysfluency in which a child has difficulty expressing himself during a period of rapid language growth.

diagnostic: An evaluation or series of tests to analyze the nature or cause of a condition.

discourse: Conversational speech.

distortion error: An articulation error characterized by a close approximation of the target sound.

dysfluency: Speech that is labored and halting, with much effort involved in verbal expression.

etiology: The cause of a given condition or difficulty.

expressive language: The ability to verbally express ideas and concepts using appropriate grammar, vocabulary, and word order. See also RECEPTIVE LANGUAGE.

fine motor skills: Skills involving use of the smaller muscles to complete a physical act (e.g., handwriting). See also GROSS MOTOR SKILLS.

fricative: A class of speech sounds formed by pushing the airstream through a constricted space or opening (e.g., "f," "v"). See also AFFRICATE, PLOSIVE.

functional: Unexplained by medical or neurological evidence.

glottis: The opening between the vocal cords.

gross motor skills: Skills involving use of the larger muscle groups to produce movement (e.g., walking). See also FINE MOTOR SKILLS.

harshness: A rough and strained vocal quality with general laryngeal tension.

hertz (Hz): The unit of measure for the frequency or pitch of sound.

hoarseness: A vocal quality that contains elements of both the harsh and breathy qualities.

hypernasality: Excessively nasal voice quality. See also HYPONASALITY.

hyponasality: Lack of sufficient nasality in the voice; similar to what the voice sounds like when a head cold is present. See also HYPERNASALITY.

incisor: One of the four front teeth in either jaw, used to cut or tear into food. See also MOLAR.

information capacity deficit: Difficulty simultaneously receiving and processing an incoming auditory message. See also AUDITORY PROCESSING DEFICIT, INTERMITTENT AUDITORY PERCEPTION, NOISE BUILD-UP, RETENTION DEFICIT, SLOW RISE TIME.

inner ear: The innermost part of the ear, responsible for balance and transmitting auditory messages to the brain. See also OUTER EAR, MIDDLE EAR, TYMPANIC MEMBRANE.

intelligibility: The clarity with which a person speaks; the ability to be clearly understood.

intensity: Loudness, measured in decibels.

intermittent auditory perception: An auditory processing deficit in which the hearing system fades in and out. See also INFORMATION CAPACITY DEFICIT, NOISE BUILD-UP, RETENTION DEFICIT, SLOW RISE TIME.

language: A means of communicating by using words or actions as symbols to denote meaning.

laryngeal: Pertaining to the larynx or voicebox.

laryngitis: An inflammation of the laryngeal area, generally including the vocal cords, characterized by a temporary loss of the voice.

linguistic: Relating or pertaining to language.

malocclusion: An improper alignment of the upper and lower set of teeth when placed in contact with each other; an abnormal bite.

mandibular: Referring to the lower jaw. See also MAXILLARY.

maxillary: Referring to the upper jaw. See also MANDIBULAR.

middle ear: The middle portion of the ear, containing tiny bones that aid in the transmission of sound from the outer ear to the inner ear. See also TYMPANIC MEMBRANE.

misarticulation: Mispronunciation of certain sounds due to improper placement of an articulator (e.g., tongue, teeth, lips).

molar: One of the teeth located in the back portion of the mouth with a rounded or flattened surface, used for chewing. See also INCISOR.

monosyllabic: Containing one syllable. See also MULTISYLLABIC.

morphology: The study of word structure or form.

multisyllabic: Containing more than one syllable. See also MONOSYLLABIC.

nasal cavity: The anatomical space above the oral cavity and behind the nose.

nasals: Sounds produced by an open nasal cavity (e.g., "m," "n," "ng").

noise build-up: A condition in which the auditory processing system breaks down if too much information is received. See also AUDITORY PROCESSING DEFICIT, INFORMATION CAPACITY DEFICIT, INTERMITTENT AUDITORY PERCEPTION, RETENTION DEFICIT, SLOW RISE TIME.

omission error: A type of articulation error in which a sound is omitted in a word.

open bite: A malocclusion in which a gap between the biting surfaces exists when the upper and lower sets of teeth are placed together.

oral cavity: The anatomical space containing the teeth, tongue, and palate.

oral-peripheral exam: An examination performed by a speech-language pathologist to assess the structure and function of the anatomical organs used to produce speech.

organic: neurological or medical in cause.

otitis media: An inflammation of the middle ear. See also patent eustachian tubes, tympanic membrane.

otorhinolaryngologist: An ear, nose, and throat specialist (ENT).

outer ear: The visible portion of the ear, the ear canal, and the eardrum, or tympanic membrane. See also INNER EAR, MIDDLE EAR, TYMPANIC MEMBRANE.

palate: The roof of the mouth, which creates a separation between the oral and nasal cavities.

patent eustachian (PE) tubes: Small plastic tubes placed within the ears if there is a threat of perforation to the eardrum, generally due to a middle ear infection.

peripheral hearing loss: A loss of hearing sensitivity in either the outer ear, middle ear, or inner ear that does not involve the central auditory processing pathways. See also CONDUCTIVE HEARING LOSS, SENSORINEURAL HEARING LOSS.

pharyngeal cavity: The anatomical space situated at the back of the oral cavity, or throat area.

phoneme: An individual sound; the smallest unit of speech.

phonology: The study of the production of sounds for speech.

pitch: The highness or lowness of a voice or other sound, measured in frequency.

plosive, or stop: Sound characterized by a temporary blockage and then release of airflow (e.g., "k," "t," "d"). Sometimes called stop. See also AFFRICATE, FRICATIVE.

pragmatics: How communication is used in a social context.

precipitating factors: Conditions that existed prior to and are at least partially responsible for the behavior occurring.

prolongation: A common behavior found in stutterers, in which the spoken word is drawn out or prolonged (e.g., "cat" becomes "caaaaaaat").

receptive language: The ability to comprehend language. See also EXPRESSIVE LANGUAGE.

repetition: A behavior common in the early stages of stuttering and in normal dysfluency characterized by repetitions of sounds, syllables, words, or phrases.

resonance: A vocal quality resulting from the vibration of several anatomical structures, especially the oral cavity and nasal cavity.

retention deficit: A condition in which auditory processing of information decreases as the length of the stimulus increases. See also AUDITORY PROCESSING DEFICIT, INFORMATION CAPACITY DEFICIT, INTERMITTENT AUDITORY PERCEPTION, NOISE BUILD-UP, SLOW RISE TIME.

schwa vowel: A weakened or neutral vowel (e.g., the first vowel in the word "among") common in stuttering moments, primarily repetitions.

secondary symptoms: Symptoms accompanying a particular behavior (e.g., facial grimacing accompanying stuttering).

semantics: The vocabulary or meanings used in language.

semivowel, or glide, or liquid: A sound characterized by a gliding motion of the articulators used to produce speech (such as "w" or "y").